Without the diligent reading, informed comment and supportive enthusiasm of Francis Adam, Gill Atkins, Alec Payne, Julian Rogers and Bruce White, this text would never have been completed and published.

Permission was sought, and generously given, to use the actual experience of real people in the process of exploring the landscapes of personality disorder. The accounts of those experiences are reproduced as faithfully as possible during the course of this narrative, although some names and details have been changed where necessary, in order to preserve anonymity.

This book is dedicated to our dear Narcissists and to those who have sustained us as we learn to move beyond them.

PREFACE

La Belle Dame Sans Merci by John Keats

(Written in 1819)

I

Oh what can ail thee, knight-at-arms,
Alone and palely loitering?
The sedge has withered from the lake,
And no birds sing.

II

Oh what can ail thee, knight-at-arms,
So haggard and so woe-begone?
The squirrel's granary is full,
And the harvest's done.

III

I see a lily on thy brow,
With anguish moist and fever-dew,
And on thy cheeks a fading rose
Fast withereth too.

IV

I met a lady in the meads,
Full beautiful - a faery's child,
Her hair was long, her foot was light,
And her eyes were wild.

V

I made a garland for her head,
And bracelets too, and fragrant zone;
She looked at me as she did love,
And made sweet moan.

VI

I set her on my pacing steed,
And nothing else saw all day long,
For sidelong would she bend, and sing
A faery's song.

VII

She found me roots of relish sweet,
And honey wild, and manna-dew,
And sure in language strange she said -
'I love thee true'.

VIII

She took me to her elfin grot,
And there she wept and sighed full sore,
And there I shut her wild wild eyes
With kisses four.

IX

And there she lulled me asleep
And there I dreamed - Ah! woe betide! -
The latest dream I ever dreamt
On the cold hill side.

X

I saw pale kings and princes too,
Pale warriors, death-pale were they all;
They cried - 'La Belle Dame sans Merci
Hath thee in thrall!'

XI

I saw their starved lips in the gloam,
With horrid warning gaped wide,
And I awoke and found me here,
On the cold hill's side.

XII

And this is why I sojourn here
Alone and palely loitering,
Though the sedge is withered from the lake,
And no birds sing.

CHAPTER ONE

The journey begins

To the south of Selborne, in the county of Hampshire, England, lies an iron water trough with a lion's face on the panel above it. The lion's face had been designed to portray a kindly look. This was surely appropriate since a generous stream of clear water gushed from its mouth into the horse trough below. The stream was known to flow reliably, even in periods of drought. Over the centuries, many a tired horse and its rider must have been grateful for the benevolence of such provision.

As the two women drove past the trough, they were starting a journey which would cover five hundred miles. It was a grey August morning and they were neither tired nor thirsty but they noticed the roadside watering spot nonetheless because of its elegant construction, and because of the gush of white water which stood out against its iron surround within the shadowed bank.

They did not know the name of the spring that Saturday morning, but a subsequent Google search by one of them later revealed that the lion provides the mouth of Wellhead Stream. Alex had had to smile when she saw that name on the screen. Talk about appropriate symbolism! There they were that Saturday morning, setting off on a journey with two heads which were very far from well. They hadn't quite thought of it in those terms but it could be said that they were indeed on a Well Head quest.

They were suffering from the same condition, Jenny and Alex, but they had not met in treatment. A series of coincidences in their lives which they had gradually unearthed over the last fifteen years had led them to a tentative friendship and then, much later, to realise that they were, in fact, similarly afflicted.

They were fundamentally 'Un Well'. The condition was a more severe attack of a previous bout from which they had both suffered, again coincidentally, in their 20's, long before they had known one another. Now in their 50's, this second affliction was more intense and their recovery appeared to be even more painfully slow, plagued by repeated relapses. There is not really one name for this condition, and no established medical treatment that either of them had discovered. They were both skilled at concealing outward and visible sign of this inward and spiritual malaise. So perhaps they had accidentally learnt to defend themselves against cures instead of arming themselves against the initial or subsequent infection.

How afflicted were they? It would be true to say that both their inner lives were blighted by their reworking of emotional bewilderment and devastation. Neither of them would have identified the condition as Post Traumatic Stress Syndrome, although perhaps they were on the wrong track in dismissing that possibility. Both of them believed that PTSS would necessarily entail specific triggers unexpectedly creating sudden flashbacks of earlier horror, as Catherine wheels ignited to delight children on firework night might suddenly remind their grandfather of a bygone explosive field of combat. Instead of being shell shocked, the women would both say, rather, that they themselves were somehow shells of their former selves – hollowed out, hologrammed into just an apparent version of what they once had been. They knew they were fortunate to have found a fellow sufferer who understood the condition from the inside. Some individuals, they guessed, were much less lucky. They might still be suffering in agonised isolation, with no access to even the first steps of a shared understanding. Jenny and Alex, however, could even laugh together about the awfulness of it at times. Through their mutual support, they had come to believe that they could eventually move through this state to something better.

Their mission this quiet, still morning was to revisit a rural area of Wales where Jenny had spent a weekend the previous year, attending a pottery workshop. She had boarded for the Saturday night in Bed and Breakfast accommodation where the proprietor had catered for every conceivable need of her guests, and far more besides, stretching to a tissue box in each bedroom which was encased in a cloth cover of the same elegant blue and white floral pattern as on the chintz frill round the dressing table, the cushions, the curtains and even along the edging of the starched linen pillow cases.

Jenny had breakfasted there in elaborate luxury on the Sunday morning and had found herself in private conversation with her hostess over a second cup of perfect coffee. Enough had been said for Jenny to recognise tortured isolation in a fellow sufferer, but back then, Jenny had not been fully aware of the nature of her own condition. Nothing explicit had been said between the two women about the annihilation common to both their inner worlds. It was to rectify this omission that Jenny and Alex were now setting out, aware of a sense of the utter ridiculousness of this quest, yet strangely compelled to embark upon it, nonetheless. Some of the awkwardness of the whole situation had been evident in the letter which Jenny had eventually nerved herself to send.

'Dear Annie,

I don't know whether you will recall our meeting but I came to stay at your B and B with my friend Clare in May 2005. We were visiting the Clay Art exhibition and had hoped to return again this year but unfortunately couldn't.

When I first stayed with you we talked about similar experiences you and I had had with our respective partners/ husbands and discovered that we both might have been involved with 'Narcissists'.

The reason for this letter is because I would like to book 2 rooms again (or the twin-bedded room) – this time for my friend Alex Thomas and myself and we are hoping you may be able to spend some time talking with us. Alex is also a 'survivor' and through our talks together and the research we have gathered, I find that I am beginning to get a better handle on my past relationships with Narcissistic men.

We are attempting to write a full length story of particular interest to survivors of dysfunctional relationships. Alex thinks that little of this nature has been published in Britain (though plenty has in America). It would really help us if we could talk with you about your experiences, feelings and coping strategies – what you told me at the time made a lasting impression on me. Of course anything you told us would be kept anonymous and any use of it would be entirely subject to your approval.

We do hope you might be able to agree to our rather strange request and perhaps you could suggest a date convenient to yourself and when your rooms are available. For us, sometime from 12th July to 15th, or at the beginning of August would be great (apart from 17th July or 4th August) but we would fit in with whatever best suited you.

I look forward to hearing from you.

With very best wishes,
Jenny Allen'

The most recent email response to this initiating missive of Jenny's lay on the dashboard in front of the passenger seat, weighed down by her glasses case.

'HELLO JENNY,

Sorry to have been so long replying. Looking forward to seeing you both on 12th August.

Directions: From Ruthin take the B5105. Follow signs towards Denbigh. Texaco garage on left. Turn left, road swings sharply right, this is the B5105. Go straight on at "T" junction. Carry straight on straight over mini roundabout heading for Cerrigydrudion, road starts to narrow and you begin to climb. Church on your right as you go round sharp bend. Black Swan pub on left. Turn second left after the pub. Carry on up the hill until you reach a signpost saying 2 ½ miles to Clogaeenog. Carry on until you drop down into the village. Turn left opposite the village hall. A few yards down on the left is a white double garage with a yellow gate in front of it, and you'll see the house sign 'Daydreams' on the top bar, with the notice about accommodation available to the right, on the corner wall of the house. YOU'VE ARRIVED!

Do you want an evening meal with me (any special dietary requirements?) Or do you want to go up the pub in the next village? At some stage, a friend of mine, Bianca, would like to meet you, if that was okay. Let me know ASAP. Many thanks.   Annie'

The printout somehow gave credence to their venture, although nothing in their hostess's wording implied much more than a business arrangement for the forthcoming Saturday night stay. So, armed with this brief confirmation of their quixotic quest, they left the gushing spring behind them. Jenny drove on through the village towards Alton, passing the single field of lavender, half cropped at this stage of the year.

"Can't you smell it?" asked Jenny.

Alex sniffed towards her window but she smelt no fragrance whatsoever. She was surprised that Jenny could, as the field was on the passenger side of the road, not the driver's. It must have been a momentary whiff which Jenny had caught from the dashboard ventilator on her side; perhaps she herself had been exhaling at the time.

"No, I can't," replied Alex, snuffling in Jenny's direction.

"Oh, *I* could."

Alex looked across at Jenny, head slightly tilted.

"It's a good smell outdoors, isn't it? It's funny that it doesn't work so well as perfume, because it just isn't sexy, somehow. Is that an image thing, do you think?"

"Yes, maybe. I suppose there's an idea about it being old ladies who like lavender," replied Jenny. "But classic perfumes like Chanel are still marketed as sexy, aren't they? And some perfumes like White Linen and Tweed actually trade on old fashioned images…."

"Would you choose a perfume with a name like that, though, if you were buying it? I wouldn't!"

"No, I don't think I would. But I'd never buy myself perfume anyway. That's the kind of thing you want to have bought for you isn't it?"

"Yes, I agree. Did Ricky ever buy you perfume?"

"No; he tended to buy much more quirky, 'chosen for me' things." Jenny's tone was nostalgic. "He was very good at that.... and the little surprise poems slipped into my purse or under my pillow, especially intimate in their delightful personal touches. It dumbfounded me that someone could love me enough to find such imaginative ways to reach my heart."

"That's so enchanting, isn't it?" mused Alex. "Marcus wasn't one for that sort of thing at all. He did buy me perfume, duty free, I suppose, coming back from lecturing abroad. Come to think of it, once it *was* White Linen. I was amazed by such sophisticated generosity, but that was only at the start of things, in my first year of working for him."

There was a pause as both women briefly recalled romantic gestures experienced in the past. When Jenny spoke again, it was with a slight lifting of her shoulders.

"Funny how even when men smell good from aftershave or something, I don't think I like that. I'd rather they didn't smell noticeably of anything bought."

"Marcus always smelt subtly expensive but I don't know what of; undoubtedly not of Old Spice or Brut, which were the only aftershaves I knew of in my youth."

Jenny smiled as she negotiated a roundabout and took the second exit. She was a confident driver, assured of the route, and at this early stage of the journey she had no need to consult the map. She let her mind retrieve a set of early images in her romance with her first great love, Joe, checking for the scents of the Sixties, while Alex was recalling with a familiar shaft of pain the contrast between the past times of receiving White Linen and the white-out of her present days.

She knew that pain well. It was a feeling like having grazed your knee, but here somehow it was the core of you that had been grazed. It was located somewhere in the middle of your stomach but yet often referred to as 'the heart'. She wondered yet again what purpose the grazed feeling served, and whether the pain could be interrupted through her own choice, rather than simply diminished temporarily, from time to time, through distraction. She thought of all the material she had read which had sometimes lightened her mind a little, but had not affected this entrenched gut feeling of desolation. It was, she reflected, perhaps a question of hitting the spot rather than spraying the target, as she seemed to be doing so obsessively. She had laboured through a stack of information sources in her research over the last three years, and wherever she read, the occasional phrase or paragraph here or there would provide a momentary glimpse of relief before becoming buried beneath further onslaughts of conceptual cure seeking.

She would often replay muddled memories of one or another research pathway over to herself, and occasionally, a shaft of gold would suddenly ignite the gloom, only to disappear just as suddenly when she attempted to focus on it. A lecture would rehearse itself in her mind, peppered with all the woeful, half digested terminology which betrays a lay reader's ignorance of the subject. She smiled sadly to herself, glancing out at pale beige fields to the left, laid bare and patterned by the undulating stripes of early harvesting.

'Ascending the Snakes and Descending the Ladders: an Examination of the Causes and Consequences of Relationship Dysfunction.

Thank you very much for that far too generous welcome to me, a complete amateur in your very distinguished field. I would like to start my talk by expressing my gratitude for being given this opportunity to address the International Forum of Relationship Disorder at their Rome Symposium. Naturally enough, the sight of the Coliseum from these magnificent windows reminds me of the plight of some unfortunate captives, many centuries ago, being faced with lions, but my situation here today seems entirely different. Here, by way of contrast, the lions of your Society have not only promised not to maul me, they have actually invited me to join them in a sumptuous picnic where ideas, rather than blood, will be generously flowing round for all to share! So thanks to this generous gesture of inclusion, I now have the temerity to approach the table, hoping for your tolerance about what little I have to bring to the feast, in this two part lecture.

My friend told me recently about childhood experiences which had been seared into her memory. When her unpredictable mother lost her temper with Laura, she would grasp hold of her little daughter's arm and leg, stand with own her legs firmly positioned apart, lean her powerful torso back and then swing and slam the child's body sideways into the kitchen wall, time after time. When she eventually ran out of breath, she would release her hold, lower the child back onto the floor and react with surprise to her daughter's tear streaked face and gulping sobs.

'Why're you cryin'?' she would enquire, with genuine curiosity. 'They don't cry in the cartoons.'

Some people see others only in cartoon form, rather than as flesh and blood. It is as if the other is unconsciously selected as a vehicle for their particular use or image, rather than as a real person with his/her own thoughts and feelings. The origins of this outlook are far from clear, but it is necessary to discount some causes of marked non social functioning from consideration here. People who suffer from neurological malfunction such as degenerative brain disease, or from a head injury, or from other specific types of brain damage may sometimes appear to treat others with total disregard. However, they will not be locked into a performance cycle which often involves grooming, targeting, destabilising and/or discarding another for their own particular purposes. This fixed inability to empathise with the targeted supplier seems to reside somewhere in the personality of certain individuals. It is very difficult to determine whether their consistently exploitative interactions may have emerged as the result of a specific cause, such as a hostile environment, a coercive collusion with an ab/user who has become the driving operational force for the duo, a deliberately chosen mode of interaction, or any combination of these or other factors.

There are various descriptors which may be applied to people who target other human beings as objects of supply. Some of these terms reflect a semi neutral, diagnostic stance. They might therefore be chosen by those exploring the topic without, as it were, an axe to grind. Available terms of this sort include, 'the self absorbed', 'non socials', 'non reciprocals' and 'stuck defenders'. The disadvantage of employing such terminology is that the descriptors sound awkward and fall between two stools. They do not strike a chord for the interested reader, and they are not, I suspect, common parlance among my distinguished audience.

I have identified a group of terms which border on sounding indulgent. The use of these words might initially appear helpful because the terms often convey the charisma and magnetism of many expediency focused operators. I refer to a group of labels such as, 'adventurers, players, pirates, pretenders, mimics and charmers'. The danger in their usage is that the implicit indulgence may serve to endorse manipulative deception, rather than simply to identify it.

Would it be wiser, then, to employ terminology with which professionals in the field are familiar? The problem here lies in the fact that not all experts accept the concept of 'personality disorder', let alone its subdivision into two toned labels such as Narcissistic, Histrionic or Borderline, to name but three. (I call them 'two toned' because they have a specific function within the DSM – 1V, that great source of diagnostic and statistical expertise about Mental Disorders, but they are also adjectives in general use which may serve as casual descriptors for people who preen themselves a lot, 'go ballistic' or 'lose it' quite often.) Even words which sound like more neutral descriptors such as, 'anti social', 'sociopath' and 'psychopath' can be very misleading. This is because tabloid and celluloid sensationalism have lifted such words beyond their etymology (antagonistic towards others, damaged socially, damaged in the mind) and brought them closer to denoting vicious thugs and murderous maniacs.

Many pejorative terms have been applied to those who cannot maintain intimate relationships with other human beings without eventually pulling them under a pathological form of overt or covert control. It is very easy to come up with a sample list here: 'users, abusers, fraudsters, offenders, controllers, perpetrators, predators, exploiters, impostors, vampires and evil people' – to name but a few! Whatever label may be employed, we are talking of those whose personality is not anchored within the grounded norms of reciprocal connection among significant others; it is 'non secured'.

So where does that leave me as I start this lecture, wishing to explore the nature of relationship dysfunction? If I cannot even decide on what terminology to use, I am not going to get very far, am I? I could 'play safe' by frequently using phrases like 'somewhere along the spectrum' when I am talking about aspects of mental health and disorder, and that would be useful in its message that it is all too 'normal' to be neurotic, or to be defensive, or to play roles which are not reflective of our true selves. We can all behave in these – and many other – psychologically unhealthy ways, according to the demanding situations in which we find ourselves. However, to sprinkle important caveats about spectrum location among all the observations to come in this lecture would inevitably result in the sort of repetition which is both irritating and distracting for an audience.

Nevertheless, it is 'sprinkling' which I shall go with, though not of provisos. I can only hope that my listeners will accept my scattering of terminology throughout this lecture. I shall be using words from the lists above, somewhat in the manner that an amateur cook might shake a jar of mixed herbs over a casserole, hoping to provide additional flavour without offending anyone's taste too much.

It is usually assumed that non reciprocal people, who may use stealth and deceit with great ingenuity, know that their interactions may leave agonised bewilderment in their wake. This presumed knowledge of theirs leads many an observer to conclude that perpetrators must therefore intend to cause enduring distress to some others in the way that they do. An assumption of this sort is often reinforced by the perception that ab/users are not apparently suffering from cognitive impairment. If we were to assess them on some well known model of personality such as the Myers Briggs Type Indicator, their preferred facets of personality would not signal any obvious dysfunction.

Using this particular fourfold indicator of cognitive functioning, ab/users appear to have unimpaired access to choices about where to direct their energies: towards the outer or the inner world, towards observable facts or new possibilities, towards logical decision making or conclusions which are belief based, and towards planning to be organised or going with the flow. They do not seem to have a handicap in mental functioning, and are generally judged by others to be 'sane', since they do not come across as severely irrational or delusional. Any marked defects in their ability to analyse, consider and reflect on an emotional level may not be at all apparent in their general interactions with another. Some of them even perform at their best in extremely complex social situations. They can treat people of personal, social or professional importance to them with consistent consideration and respect. It is easy to conclude that in their abusive relationships, they must be making a deliberate choice to be harmful, once they have managed to establish a sufficient level of power and control over their target. The recurrent verdict on these offenders is that they could evidently moderate their unfeeling behaviour towards another, if they wanted to.

There is an Irish phrase, referring to those professional music makers who delight local audiences with their lilting violin melodies but are, in fact, cruel deflators at home; 'the sort who leaves his fiddle at the door.' The image here is of the musical instrument being deliberately put down on the threshold of the home, emphasising the element of conscious choice in the positioning.

So c/harmers are often judged harshly by those few detached observers who are able to pinpoint what they are doing to their victims. It is presumed that the perpetrators' ability to process their own emotions is unimpaired, since their other analytical skills seem to be firmly in place. However, it might be simplistic to assume that people's powers of emotional empathy generally develop according to the culturally accepted norm. The guiding principle which most authentically sociable people come to regard as self evident is, 'Don't do as you would not be done by'. It is inexplicable to such people that this tenet could ever be totally disregarded by others within their own networks. Even quite young children splutter with righteous indignation if a player breaks the rules of a board game, despite the fact that the cheating does no actual damage to others in the context of family entertainment.

In common with all other human beings, adults who are c/harmers will inevitably encounter slices of misfortune for which they are unprepared. Their response to these unnerving events, which lie beyond their control, tends to stray beyond the perceived limits of 'loss management'. Instead, they skip the, 'Don't do as you would not be done by' principle, and respond instantly from their poised emergency defence mode. Whether this mode employs the softest variety of passive aggression or ruthless combative onslaught, or a complex combination of both, the underlying intention will be Self Preservation at all costs. In their subsequent behaviours, they turn out to be moving up the Snakes and down the Ladders, although they may well deceive the observer by pausing when their direction of movement is under observation.

Those with keen enough eyes to spot the simulation, however, are often, like children, scarcely able to contain their indignation at this emotional cheating by the offender. Observers and victims often become enmeshed in reiterating the rules of the human interaction game obsessively, unable to come to terms with the fact that the offending player is not abiding by them. But could it be that, back in early childhood, the chemical and electrical circuits within the offenders' infant brains have become impaired, and the consequent malfunctioning eventually results in a radically different code of interactive behaviour from that of the supposedly functional majority? If so, why and how might this have come about?

It is tempting to say that it all comes down to anti social genetic traits. After all, covert or overt abuse of power appears to pass down through one generation to the next, whether in family, social or inter/national networks. However, this theory can be countered by the evident disparity in social ability and emotional stability between children who are all offspring of the same mother and father. If it were a simple matter of inherited genes, each child of well adjusted, sociable parents would be likely to display those same desirable personality traits. Similarly, all the children born of the corrosive union between two psychologically damaged adults would bear the burden of that genetic disadvantage.

This is plainly not the case. One (or more) child in a family where all the children appear to be warmly nurtured in a benevolent setting may develop inflexibly (passive) aggressive, self promoting traits while his brothers and sisters, apparently experiencing the same household and parenting, do not. Correspondingly, infant offspring of severely delinquent parents who are removed from their family of origin and settled within healthier families in infancy have been tracked through adolescence into maturity, and deemed eventually to have 'made it' as authentic, connected members of society. A supportive environment provided for them in their adoptive family from a very early age can thus, apparently, outweigh the theoretic disadvantage of their genetic inheritance. Even those children who are born of two violent parents and raised in an atmosphere of extreme hostility may, somehow or other, be able to overcome this inauspicious start in life, and go on to flourish in positive relationships which they forge within a variety of circles.

Is it possible to identify the mysterious ingredients at work here — those 'somehow or other' elements? Let us start with a relatively accessible group of determining factors. Each infant's experience of growing up in the same household can be markedly different. These variations include the mother's physical, medical and psychological state during her child's gestation months in the womb, the process of birth itself, earliest bonding between caregiver and child, birth order, gender, family size and dynamics during the infant's crucial time of early development. What the infants have in common, however, is that their extremely pliable brains are being honed by these variations, for better or for worse, in patterns which are likely to be enduring. This is because the quality of care which an infant receives during the vital first three years of life will affect the actual size and structure of the infant's *developing brain, the electro chemistry of her/ his mental circuits.*

Also of essential relevance at this stage – and during the next years of young life – are particular external circumstances such as economic/social disruption affecting the provision of food and shelter, and other hazards such as family break up or bereavement, as well as the network of friends, early school companions, teachers and other relevant adults which the individual child encounters over time. In even the most challenging of childhoods, it could be that one positive incident or a fortuitous combination of such circumstances enabled one child in the family to escape potential long term insecurity of attachment.

Among other important variants which may imperceptibly shape a child's psychological development is the weight of certain expectations which may be laid, consciously or unconsciously, on the minor by his or her elders. If two major caregivers are present, there may be contrasting responses to the child's placement in age among siblings, for example. Each parent (or parent substitute) might unconsciously project his or her own childhood experience or observations of being an only child, or of being the middle child, onto their only offspring or onto their second child of three. These parental projections, often in stark contrast to one another, can have a profoundly formative impact on the infant's psychological development, despite the fact that none of the family is consciously aware of any of them.

The projections – which may, of course, also be displayed by other family members such as a resentful older brother or an overbearing grandmother – could be triggered by any number of unconscious interpretations about the new arrival's impact on their lives, all of which actually stem from expectations linked with the projectors' own life experiences. Among these unfounded interpretations could be conclusions about the infant offspring's perceived temperament. This concept may include the degree to which the infant appears to reach out or withdraw in response to its immediate environment.

While some aspects of the infant's psychological individuality may indeed be genetically predetermined, it is probable that adult caregivers and/or other family members will develop their own preconceived notions about an infant's characteristics, and respond to the child accordingly. Habitual initiatives and responses may gradually become a set pattern between family member and minor, regardless of the unrecognised source of this feedback loop. There are much greater opportunities for spontaneous creativity within the loop when the origin of the patterned relationship interplay is, by way of contrast, based on an alert awareness of the individual child's current signals and a sensitively attuned response to them as they arise. When this is the case, the child has a better chance of developing a secure inner sense of Self within the first years of life. In even the most apparently healthy and 'successful' of families, however, this is by no means always what happens.

If the child has a parental figure who has, in painful circumstances, departed from the family group, there is likely to be a crucial impact from that very absence. One of many relevant factors in this impact is the remaining caregiver's attitude to the unavailable co parent. This may well involve projections foisted on the child, such as the presumed requirement for overprotection or compensation (applied either to the child or to the remaining parent or both) or for controlling vigilance lest the infant has the potential to develop any perceived faults of the absent parent. Sanctification of the missing adult and the resultant pressure on the child to live up to this idealisation is an example of the opposite sort of projection. All of these unrealistic expectations may distort the infant's developing capacity to attune his own needs creatively to those of others around him who regularly play a part in his nurturing environment.

It becomes apparent that determining how and why a fixed hostile defence against others may become established in the very young child is an extremely complex matter. How much easier it would be if we could just declare that psychological dysfunction which goes against the accepted cooperative norms of the society is down to our genes, the replicators within us, rather than environmental influences! Yet a moment's thought allows us to see that on-going replication of those genes depends on flexibility and adaptability to ever changing conditions around us. Each *generation in every human society throughout the world needs to register these changes and to shape the development of their own infants' neurological pathways in order to meet the demands which inconstant conditions will make of them in their turn. Caregivers have a unique opportunity to shape this potential fitness for adaptive purpose during their infants' earliest years, but each society may provide either support or sabotage of this nurturing process to varying degrees.*

If the healthy development of the infant brain has been effectively sabotaged, the young child will be unresponsive to gradual learning about cooperative socialisation within the group. This sort of emotional intelligence is hard won, involving delayed gratification and longer term objectives, and relying on shared notions of guilt, responsibility and sympathetic awareness. The child's distorted psychological makeup, acquired predominately through a sustained lack of two way bonding in infancy, will be no choice of his own. He learns to maintain a rigid form of defence, which is brought into being by the need to shore up a fragile self constructed identity. This hypervigilant, defensive self has had to be fashioned from within for survival in a psychological mine field.

The actively non social child consequently loses out on the manifold family opportunities to develop authentic human connection, year on year. The resulting incremental damage forms an invisible barrier against acceptance within the group. Not only will he be unable genuinely to participate in the group's cooperative interactions but, sooner or later, he is likely to be subject to the group's avoidance or condemnation of him — a judgement made by the majority of the group who are not similarly disadvantaged — for failing to develop a quintessential authenticity. Sensing this condemnation, the non social individual may reinforce his already rigid defence system to shore up his emotional detachment from those whom he perceives as hostile others.

The holding of an entrenched hostile defensive position against others in the group is counter productive for the individual, even if s/he successfully conceals this exhausting psychological stance. This is because s/he can never relax enough to benefit from spontaneous, creative interchanges with others. More fortunate group members have gradually learnt to participate in an increasing number of interactive feedback loops. These vital circuits of human connection modify and expand the inner reality of those who operate, to some degree at least, in emotional free space. At best, we enter into a constant process of dynamic interchanges, allowing us opportunities throughout our lives to mourn, soothe and rejoice for ourselves and for others. To be denied access to this process is an enduring tragedy for any individual, even if s/he has no idea of the deprivation or its significance.

I would now like to consider the impact of an individual's fixed defensive stance on the group as a whole. Many of those who consider themselves active members of a community would agree that behaviour which results in an illegal violation of another's rights should be prohibited, in order to preserve the safety of the group as a whole. Punishment may succeed in acting as a deterrent, but even if it does not, it serves to enforce the expectation of cooperative behaviour in the group.

However, exploitative people often violate the rights of another in a way which escapes detection and would not be punishable by law, even if it was possible to prove the violation. It is impossible for the State to legislate effectively against the breaking of a cherished personal promise, or of a heart, particularly when the victim's hurt is all on the inside and cannot easily be demonstrated to the eyes of the world. So how is such a victim to have any redress against invisible yet devastating injury? The group bases its core stability on the idea that those who offend its laws will be called to account. This means that the wounded victim naturally feels entitled to such justice if s/he has been the target of profoundly damaging personal offence. At the very least, the 'better nature' of the offender must be called into play, and remorse needs to be evident if any sort of closure is to be obtained for the injured party.

But if the overreaching drive of the ab/user is to be armed against others, then the capacity for guilt, shame, sympathy and love will be stunted. Without these 'secondary' (learnt) emotions, which most infants gradually pick up through responding intuitively to the cues of the loving caregivers around them, the socially unresponsive child is left with a predominance of the primary emotions which do not require socialisation to develop. These emotions are sometimes labelled 'primary' because they are the 'Flight or Fight' responses such as fear, anger and disgust, which predate human evolution. Other primary responses such as surprise, anticipation and satisfaction are on tap when the need to confront or escape dies down. Empathy for those they have wounded and remorse for the harm done are secondary emotions which ab/users seldom have at their disposal.

Many thousands of years ago, when group living for the majority of people on our earth was based on survival against the odds, emergency signals about Flight or Fight had to be transmitted urgently to kin through body movement and audible/visible expression of incipient danger. These signals were instinctive reactions to a major threat and their message would pass instantaneously to all those within range of the warning.

The world we live in today still provides many stressful crises of Fight or Flight which cause our bodies to go on physical alert, and we still experience a chemical rush when this happens, although individual levels of physiological awareness may vary considerably. However, communicating adults in a stable social environment – whether at work or in the home – generally avoid employing the resultant flood of extra energy for forceful physical combat or for actual rushed departure from the scene. Our immediate responses may be demonstrated through our facial expressions and body language, but as our social interactions have become more complex, we have developed more subtle ways of managing our reactive emotions.

These responses will more often be contained through words, whether voiced externally or internally. In order to dissolve the internalised stress we have accumulated in such a crisis, we need to become aware of the emotions which are attached to it, and to seek an authentic way to accommodate or move beyond them within ourselves. This capacity first to reflect on our own emotional response provides us with a range of choices for our consequent interactions with others. We can develop skills focused on whether and how to express our responses appropriately and effectively to those around us, and to allow them to do the same.

This expansion and refinement of signaling within the group allows today's members to learn to 'read' one another accurately without an instant resort to extreme reactions, and to become socially cohesive, whether in times of danger or tranquillity. We need to be able to interpret the emotions of other group members in order to exchange coded warnings of incipient external threats, and to cooperate at maximum efficiency in challenging environments. These threats and challenges may be very different from those which faced our ancestors long ago, but we still need support and cooperation in our daily lives in order to deal with them.

Those people who are actively non social — who are anarchic in terms of authentic collaboration with others — will be unable to deal with stress through internal processing and subsequent communication of genuine emotion. They may instead constantly seek to create a psychologically unstable environment around them, in order to acclimatise their external ambiance to their sustained inner Flight or Fight readiness. (If the atmosphere around them was generally serene and harmonious, it would serve to point up their inappropriate level of vigilance, and tend to 'blow their cover'.) The red alerted Self might provide protection for them but it denies them access to the sort of intuitive education which the group as a whole may take for granted. Members of their circle may sometimes be puzzled by the responses of stuck defenders, but they tend wrongly to assume that the non secured individual (who may present herself as being very secure indeed!) naturally has the same adaptive inner processes as functional others do. This assumption vastly increases the confusion and bewilderment of those group members who subsequently feel their trust has been betrayed.

The victims who are left floundering in the wake of abusive relationships have often been 'strung along' by plausible transactions which mask actual emotional disconnection. Without these perfected techniques, the pretender's marginalisation from his particular supply group might gradually be increased in a vicious circle of alienation. One of many strategies he may employ is to imitate or borrow the openly connected behaviour of functioning people around him. Ironically, this psychological filching of his may serve to create a sense of 'soul mate' synchronicity with him, in the mind of a potential victim. It is virtually impossible for a fellow group member to distinguish between genuine human interconnection and what is actually an expedient appropriation of this behaviour, a type of performance which has often been polished by long term imitative practice.

I turn to the words of a victim who eventually came to recognise this psychological infestation for what it was:

'Of course she endorsed my deepest truths and shared every aspect of my value system – she lifted them from me and ran with them in the most exhilarating way! I felt treasured and cocooned from the inside out, as if my whole being was surrounded by the warmest and gentlest of light. I thought she was illuminating me but actually, she was just mirroring some little inner light of mine, doubling it through reflecting it back at me. When she had used up all my shining, I was left in the bleakest of darkness while she moved on merrily to appropriate another source of borrowed radiance.'

These words might tempt one to rephrase that old observation, 'Imitation is the sincerest form of flattery' into an updated warning: 'Psychological imitation is the most dangerous form of flattery, if it means that exploitation is mistaken for sincerity'.

Relationship dysfunction can severely distort healthy family life, generation on generation. It impairs the establishment of mutual supportive networks within the family and beyond it. Those who have suffered at the hands of non social entrepreneurs are often profoundly traumatised. Whole swathes of people in some societies at certain epochs may actually be exterminated at the hands of an exploitative individual who has obsessively employed his charismatic powers of leadership to achieve the ultimate control (life or death) over those he dominates.

At first, then, it seems hard to imagine any possible

contribution to the group from those members who apparently have a chronic lack of sensitively-attuned social awareness. However, their corresponding surfeit of aggression, competitiveness and need for control, along with their Flight or Fight primary emotions, may be channelled into the sort of single minded, obsessive activity which can be of outstanding benefit to society in general, if not to those individuals who attempt to connect with them on a personal level. Not all brilliant entrepreneurs are devoted spouses or popular contributors to the group in their lifetime, however significant their contributions may eventually be to the advancement of progress in their field. As Aquinas would have it, 'Etiam peccata' which roughly translates into, 'Even dysfunction can indirectly benefit society"!

There is a second possible contribution which we might consider. Perhaps, in certain circumstances, there can be a vital place for undermining or attacking from within the group itself. This could serve to stimulate group members urgently to improve their communications with one another, to question the hierarchies operating within the group, and ultimately, to review the very foundations upon which the community rests.

Thirdly, some non social mavericks, once they gain physical maturity, may choose to exploit other group members sexually, resulting in an increased number of offspring conceived with a variety of partners. This random element and its disruptive effect upon the group's culturally dictated habits of procreation may make an essential contribution to the adaptability of future generations. It may serve to counter a tendency towards inbreeding within the group, where courtship may generally be influenced by stereotypical attitudes about choice of mate. Too much dominance over mating choices within the group's culture may result in future generations of children inheriting a highly concentrated set of genetic traits; a shallow and confined gene pool. Given that the ultimate rationale for our existence is for our genes to make their way down the generations, and that this is facilitated by the emergence over time of adaptive design features, it would appear to be highly advantageous to widen the range of genetic building blocks available.

Thus, there could be both individual and group benefits in the existence of a 'wild card' element — a tiny minority who provide the tangy element of deceit or a sharp spice of betrayal which runs counter to the cultural and social norms of the majority. It is important to remember, of course, that throughout history there have been societies where aggressive behaviour has become essential for survival and has become the norm within that particular culture. In these situations, past, present and future, it may eventually turn out to be the 'wild card' element of decency which puts an individual out of kilter with those who surround him. Such totalitarian groups may well achieve considerable success in terms of unchallenged power and control over their own members and, in time, over other communities as well. However, dictators often come to overestimate their capacity for control by expanding their boundaries of operation too far. This eventually results in the downfall of the society as a whole, leaving the remaining individuals caught up in a raw, brutish struggle for short term individual survival.

It is not generally easy to determine whether decency or exploitation is the majority's social norm within any one community. One can only surmise that in groups where cooperative and mutually supportive behaviour appears to be the dominant mode of interaction, the earliest child rearing practices which have been established over time are more likely to have been beneficial for the healthy development of the infants' brains. This vital nurturing period would involve a 'good enough' response to infant needs on a sustained basis, incorporating the emotional feedback loop of empathetic fine tuning between caregiver and infant. In societies where relationship bonding and mutually supportive lifestyles are seen as essential, this sort of infant care within an extended family is likely to be fostered by the group, generation upon generation.

Looking back into the group systems of the past, it would appear that hunter gatherer communities may have fostered their young towards psychological health, however harsh their physical environment might have been. Infants brought up in developing societies which are still agrarian appear to start life harmoniously contained in their carers' working and resting routines, with the baby's attachment often firmly put in place by actual binding close up to his mother's body. However, over the centuries, developing societies have tended to move towards more urban environments. This has had an increasing impact on how infants' earliest routines of care have become regimented to fit into more exacting schedules and labour demands. In these more complex societies, the sensitive rearing of infants may not be regarded as a high priority in the society's drive for progress as a whole.

It is no surprise here if the pressure of responding intuitively to infant need may fall heavily on one poorly supported caregiver or on alternating part time substitutes. Positive feedback loops between essential caregiver and infant are less likely to be the norm in societies where economic well being is the highest priority and where earning power is generally given greater emphasis than psychological health. Back in Elizabethan times, the Londoner Orlando Gibbons, composing his Silver Swan madrigal, may be writing of what he perceives as a general deterioration in people's character. Perhaps this pessimistic view reflects the rising predominance of city life and court power in a new age of expansion, a change which might well adversely affect the more intuitive child rearing practices of lost rural communities. The dying swan laments,

'Farewell, all joys! O Death, come close mine eyes!
More Geese than Swans now live, more Fools than Wise.'

In this lecture, I have been attempting to see the pathologically exploitative individual in the context of his upbringing, and also in terms of his impact upon the more closely associated members of his containing circles, as well as on the group as a whole. A compassionate and cohesive society seeks to establish a stable and stimulating environment for the next generations, intending to decrease the incidence of pathological defences and destructive behaviours within the population. One increasingly endorsed strategy to achieve this aim is to provide the best possible information, support and resources for those who nurture infants into childhood and beyond it.

What help is available in our society for those who have already grown into adulthood as abusers of power, and for those who become their victims? As far as the exploiters are concerned, the main problem lies in the fact that those who constantly operate without empathy are extremely unlikely to be aware of the profound significance of this deficiency, and to seek any sort of help. They do not have access to those core feelings of empowerment and self worth which are primarily established during infancy. Over time, well adapted people constantly fine tune their innate need for power and recognition within the group, seeking new ways to feel at ease within their ever changing networks. This ongoing process of refinement remains beyond the reach of the disordered. The inevitable result is a distortion in their sense of Self. A healthy self empowerment becomes instead a pathological need for control, and attuned self worth is twisted into self obsession. The obsession with Self can take the form of loathing and/or idealising one's core being.

Impostors may realise, through logical deduction, that some quality which might be tagged, 'fellow feeling' is generally regarded as a Good Thing by others around them, and that they themselves should also attempt to display behavioural evidence of this trait. They often assume that everyone else is similarly simply adopting these affirmed attributes for his/her own social advancement. Their talent for convincing displays of desirable traits, deceiving themselves just as effectively as those around them, is often considerable, since, in common with all other members, their survival depends on avoiding exclusion from the group. But the art of sustained belonging is very much more difficult for those who have, from infancy, been denied that vital, pre verbal experience of attuned feedback with a tender significant other.

Without this intuitive initiation into the experience of human connection, simulation of it becomes one obvious alternative, in order to claim a place in an interdependent group. This means that some exploiters, long skilled out of necessity in acting a part, are virtually unidentifiable as such to those who put intimate trust in them until it is too late to withdraw it. A victim is frequently left in a state of desolation, and feels as if the essence of his or her own personality has been inexplicably eradicated. If a victim eventually realises that s/he has been exploited by a pretender, s/he may be deeply traumatised because it is unthinkable to have felt deeply connected, maybe for several decades, to a long term player rather than to a genuine co participant in human relationships.

It has been said that experts make very little money treating long term performers who only have intermittent access to insight or self awareness. Professionals may occasionally be requested to step in and guide these pretenders towards a genuine need to address and move beyond their underlying vulnerabilities, but any such therapy may often be abruptly abandoned by the client if it presents any challenge to her constructed false self. Psychiatrists are instead kept profitably busy by treating numerous clients who feel they are 'losing it' at the hands of players, or clients who have lost out to them completely.

Perhaps those who have been targeted can be helped to recover if they come to see more clearly the precise nature of the game which has been played, where their own personal identity was an inappropriate stake to risk. The pretender herself will often be able to move on to an alternative (sometimes contrasting) cycle of simulation with no access to remorse or regret. However, the shattered victim needs to learn much more about the games people play, and about how exploitative players have used particular vulnerabilities of those they target to pull them into participation.

It is often the case that pretenders choose 'tenders' as targets, if I may use the latter collective word to mean those people pleasers who naturally tend to others as a way of finding meaning in their lives. To do this from a position of mental health, one must be sure to attend to one's own needs in the first place, and to be attuned to the healthiest inner option for oneself in relation to others. 'Tenders' often ignore this intuitive inner wisdom of theirs in their rush to be rescuers or maintainers. Such eager volunteers are easy targets for control and supply, thus unconsciously contributing to their own exploitation by pretenders. It is this *sort of vulnerability which the victim must, in the end, address. Yet many survivors avoid this key issue, choosing instead to maintain an obsessive dedication to healing the profound wounds of the ab/user which are, in fact, far beyond their reach. Rescuers of parasitic people need to beware of stepping into a triangular operational space, as identified by Karpman back in the Sixties; a stifling confinement which provides only two other positions available to both parties – that of victim or that of persecutor. Many rescuers find themselves stuck in a relentless routine where they apparently can't step out of this sequence of movement and keep clear of it subsequently. It is very hard for them to discard the sentimental illusion, powerfully conveyed in so much of our popular culture, that 'All you need is Love'. Not to discard it means the victim might justifiably be accused of contributory negligence.*

It may seem a daunting task for a survivor to undertake but ultimately, it is likely to be the most effective possible path towards recovery. So, as I draw my first lecture to a close, I turn my eyes again to those fine windows facing onto the Coliseum and think once more of the captives who had little hope of survival, many centuries ago, against the lions poised to tear them to pieces. Perhaps one of the underlying principles which unites us all here today is to recognise the on going psychological struggle for survival between captive and predatory human, and to seek ways of freeing them both from ever participating in such a cruel and deadly sport. '

"D'you think we're actually stark raving bonkers to be doing this, Alex?"

Jenny broke into Alex's internal monologue, posing the question with her usual abruptness. She was negotiating her entry onto the Basingstoke dual carriageway, but a familiar undercurrent of humour spilled through her words.

"It was your idea, if you remember, not mine!" Alex responded swiftly.

"Oh now, wait a minute – no way was it just my idea!"

"Jenny, I would never have proposed a trip to Wales! I'm a coward about a journey of five miles, let alone five hundred!"

"But you can deal with people; I'm scared this will all blow up in our faces when we get there!"

"How could it do that? We know Annie's expecting us, and she has a good idea why we're coming, from the letter you've sent. If she turns frosty on us, we just have a good B and B session and drive home again tomorrow. It won't be a disaster. At least we will have had this adventure together. But to me, the thought of finding my way there, and so much of it on complicated, fast moving motorways, is the ultimate nightmare."

"Well, I suppose that's why we make a good team," remarked Jenny, sounding slightly relieved. "We have complementary skills, don't you think? The driving doesn't worry me a bit, but the people bonding thing unnerves me immediately. You're the opposite."

"We're opposite in lots of ways, really. Look at how I bog things up so often, and only learn to get anything right eventually by getting it wrong repeatedly. You don't seem to operate shambolically at all. You seem to be very good at all sorts of practical things, Jenny. I mean planning, admin and all that, seeing to the detail and getting it right first time. Applying for the lottery funding for that sculpture in the quad at school, with all the hideous paperwork involved, must have been absolute hell, but you did it! Yet your art stuff is creative and spontaneous; remember that art workshop down in Devon where your papier mache ostrich stopped everyone in their tracks! That's a rare combination you know, to be sparklingly arty and dead efficient!"

"Oh, Alex, you always talk to people like this; you just play to their ears."

"No, I don't; I mean it! Anyway, it's not just me; the entire department felt the same about you. Even the three duchesses in the coffee machine corner were admirers of yours, and they are the hardest taskmasters to please. And my guarded husband, who is never quick to praise, thinks you're great! And just look at the friends you have outside school, dear Jenny! You've got mates you've known for donkey's years and gone abroad with and lived through all sorts of joys and disasters with. And there are kids, too, who write to you years after they've left school, and say that they're running an art gallery or doing an Art M.A. because of you."

"Hmpff! Well, yes, I do find those contacts from girls touching, but they are very rare, you know. Most of the time I'm just muddling through, trying to keep my nostrils above the surface of the water."

"Well, at least you managed that! I couldn't even keep treading water, could I? Invalided out of the school as a head case, and put out to grass early, at considerable expense to the poor old N.U.T.! Funny that, isn't it? The N.U.T. who pension off NUT-ter-teachers."

"But you got over it, Alex. You built up a new sort of life for yourself and you're fine now, aren't you?"

"Well, yes, but I built it on shifting sands, really, looking back on it. Dan couldn't have been a more supportive husband, and never put a foot wrong in the couple of months it took for the antidepressants to kick in to their full extent. He was never patronising, never impatient, always gently encouraging, and he never said, 'I told you so!' which he might well have done because he had warned me I was going under somehow.

"I've never really worked out quite why it had happened. I guess I'd never let myself relax while I was at work because at some level, I considered the job well beyond my level of competence. It would only be by driving myself into total overload that I might just manage to do a reasonable job. But it wasn't overwork that did for me; I suppose a number of factors came together, like doing the M.A., and my dear mum dying, and just gradually beginning to get worn down to the extent that I was getting afraid of entering the school buildings, let alone the classroom. It got to the point that my heart was pounding in terror as I walked along the corridor towards my room. I felt like some essential energy within me was just petering out, day by day, and there was nothing I could do to plug into it again.

"I suppose the antidepressants replenished the depleted chemicals, whatever they were, but by then, I'd lost confidence that I could get back my classroom stamina and resilience. Once I knew I couldn't return to teaching without a constant terror that I'd plunge down again, Dan was always trying to find ways to alleviate my self condemnation and my overwhelming guilt for having let everyone down at school, and the English Department in particular. I remember sitting at home, week after week, still with the shakes, and still noticing the lesson change times every fifty minutes and imagining some poor soul or other dealing with class after class of mine. And even now, long after most of the department has retired or moved elsewhere, I can still find our Old Bag reunions daunting because I'm so ashamed of my pathetic exit from the teaching stage, in contrast to their sensible and professional departures."

Alex grimaced in profound embarrassment at the thought. She sighed before continuing,

"Dan had got hold of the idea, from my doctor, I think, that my depression was an illness which simply needed treatment and about six months' worth of time, and he never wavered from repeating that reassurance to me. I never accepted that 'illness' concept myself, but I heard the words each time Dan said them, and was grateful for such a comforting attempt to counter my own self disgust. Dan even tore out the article in *The Guardian* for me in which a certain Professor Marcus Hilton was appealing for volunteers in a great new arts project based only a few miles from me. Ironic, really, that Dan was the instrument for my meeting Marcus in the first place!

"It wasn't long before I began working for Marcus, doing the mundane bits of research ferreting about those manuscripts; you know, that batch of nineteenth century poetry and letters which was discovered during renovations of Uplands House, but had not yet, back then, been proved to be genuine. I also worked on databases, listing countless names and addresses of the Great and the Good. These were databases which Marcus had set up, for fund raising purposes or 'schmoozing', as he called it. The job itself was hardly inspirational but he seemed to inspire me. I think I began to focus my gradual recovery more round his identity than mine. I suppose I was imprinted on him, or something.

"I knew something significant was happening but I couldn't quite work out what. I did try to describe it to Dan. I even tried to explain it, one to one, when I had the chance, to Bella and to each of the boys, right from the start. I explained that there was – er – some sort of an emotional involvement between me and my new boss. I suppose that I played it down, as a bit of a laugh, but at that stage, it really didn't seem very significant anyway. I expect they thought it was a crush, somehow connected with the loss of my teaching career or coming out of my depression or being middle aged or something. You can imagine that they weren't keen to seek further information, poor loves! Parents' emotional stuff is always so embarrassing! They were all young adults by then and had their own lives to sort out. I assured them that there was no need to worry.

"Bella didn't say so, but I could see from her face that she was very protective of her dad, and a bit anxious on his behalf. Maybe I was wrong to burden any of them but I believed that keeping secrets and telling lies was what did most harm in families. So I tried to circumvent hurt by being direct from the start.

"I actually told Dan later the very day that Marcus had suddenly proclaimed to me in his office that he 'adored me' – a favourite phrase of his – and that he feared he was falling in love with me. I told Dan that I was shocked by this and it did, indeed, take me hours to stop shaking. But I added that I supposed I loved Marcus back. I remember saying to Dan, 'I don't know what else to do when someone loves me.' Dan seemed more concerned that I was back to trembling than anything else; he was very gentle about it all. I explained the revelation as a version of courtly love from King Arthur sort of thing – you know: a lot of romantic idealisation and no sex.

"Dan didn't get the 'chivalry' bit at all, and why should he? He certainly knew romanticism wasn't his style. But he accepted that as a husband he was introverted and self contained, a man of actions rather than words, who had little dependence on me. He decided that Marcus could probably offer me diverting conversations and ideas which might fill some of the gaping void which losing my job had opened up in my life.

"Marcus's wife might have responded in the same way if Marcus had decided to tell her about it, tactfully dressed up as a meeting of minds, at that point. She was certainly intimidated by the intensely academic nature of his work, but was utterly supportive of his career. Maybe she would have been relieved that someone else was able to listen in fascination to his ruminations about the next chapter of his latest great work. It's unlikely, though, when I come to think about it. She struck me as the sort of wife who maintained the family's privacy as if it was under siege against intruders.

"Marcus could have had no doubt as to where her loyalties lay, although he did sometimes seem to resent the amount of time she spent text messaging one or other of their children. He frequently boasted about Tessa and his kids to me or to anyone else who would listen. He was particularly proud of her recent promotion to the ranks of Primary schools inspector and also of his younger son's rapid success in setting up a software business in Jersey. There seemed no question of rocking either his or my marriage, then or in the future.

"Dan accepted my word for it when I said I wasn't taking anything away from him by loving Marcus; that it was all some strange sort of lyrical game. The fact that actual sex wasn't high on the agenda, a key requirement of Courtly Love, of course, might have helped, but Dan did not seem anxious about that aspect of things. He has never been a sexually demanding or possessive man. He asked no questions about any sort of physical affection between me and Marcus. He said he didn't want to know, and I respected that."

Alex was aware that she was somehow trying to make excuses for herself as she spoke. She found it impossible to explore this topic without an underlying need for self justification. She sought for a more objective tone as she continued,

"Anyway, this imprinting thing..... . I wondered at the time whether I was somehow rebuilding a sort of identity for myself, after the breakdown, through Marcus's professed dazzling admiration for me. Little did I know then that actually, the boot was probably on the other foot; that he was building a new sort of identity for himself through my very obvious admiration of him! Certainly I was – er – what is it? 'introjecting,' I think...... that is, I was living up to his dreams of me being his possession.

"All the time, though, Jenny, I actually thought I had the measure of him, and I honestly believed that I was coming from a position of warm amusement for this smoothie academic who was so keen to establish his achievements and his sexiness in such a delightfully playful way. It came across as classic male vulnerability to me at the time, and I thought I could handle it fine."

"You must have been very flattered, surely? Wasn't it extremely good for the ego?" queried Jenny, probing gently for more honesty.

"Well, yes, I suppose so, but I didn't think I was subject to his flattery, despite the fact that he was a professor and such a successful writer and so much the focus of everyone's attention. I never believed the charming things he told me about myself, but I certainly loved to hear the words said. His pet name for me was 'Angel' because he declared that was what I was to him! I began trying to be his angelic muse because that seemed to be what he needed. But I thought it was just an indulgent role I could play towards him, the way you'd act along with a toddler's fantasies.

"He used to tell me little things about himself which indicated to me that he was a bit – er – lost, somehow. I remember he told me that a university colleague, a female academic, had once said to him, 'The trouble with you, Marcus, is that you're just a series of constructions.' He seemed very troubled about this and returned to it several times, asking me what I thought she had meant.

"There were certain lines or scenes in films which seemed to make him anxious, too. He was happier with adventure or comedy films but disquieted by films which focused on how people interacted with one another, particularly if a woman was hurt by a man's behaviour. He would puzzle about people's capacity to brutalise their loved ones mentally, and seemed to perceive women as the usual perpetrators of this sort of behaviour. He said that in his experience within the family, both in the past and in the present, he saw women constantly putting forward patient, loving explanations of a series of profound sins committed by their menfolk, especially by himself. He told me that Tessa persistently complained in this gentle way about his shortcomings. Yet he himself kept a secret journal of Tessa's transgressions in thought, word and deed, as he saw them. The sort of incidents he cited – like her not putting the vegetables out on his dinner plate but expecting him to help himself from the saucepan on the stove – seemed to me strange ones for him to take to heart, especially as he admitted that he was very quick to point out her supposed errors of speech to her face, and even her perceived social awkwardness.

"I remember on one occasion that we met, Marcus seemed particularly distressed. He had been taken aback by a funeral address given about a fellow lecturer, who had been struck down relatively early in life, leaving a widow and two teenage children. In the course of the eulogy, the dead man had been praised for the way that he would always put his work on hold if one of his children sought his company in his study. He apparently regarded their needs as first priority. Marcus remembered particularly the part of the address which stipulated that it was these incidences of generous attentiveness, rather than one's achievements in the outside world, which came to be the most treasured memories once a person had died. He puzzled about this with me, admitting sadly that his priorities would always have been exactly the opposite from his dead colleague's."

Alex glanced across at Jenny, who nodded, encouraging her to continue.

"There were lots of times when Marcus seemed genuinely confused about apparently trivial challenges. I remember once, much later on in our time together, he had been persuaded to go on some adult arts workshop one Saturday morning, as part of a fundraising project for the cathedral. (He had presented himself there as a helper soon after taking up the arts job, originally as some sort of volunteer manager of the cathedral servers, but, naturally enough, he was rapidly promoted to the Dean's right hand man, spin doctor, exhibition organiser and publicist.) Anyway, the art teacher obviously had some trendy little tasks to get the group started, one of which was to fold a page into four squares and use appropriate colours to illustrate any four different moods, in the four different spaces. I suppose most kids could do that quite easily couldn't they? Yellow for feeling sunny and happy, Red for anger.... could they?"

"Um, yes – probably they could, from seven upwards."

"Well, Marcus explained to me that he just didn't know where to start. The other half dozen adults, including Tessa, completed the task within the couple of minutes allocated, before he had even put crayon to paper. He said he got a bit wound up when he realised that he was the only one who found the exercise difficult. The workshop leader noticed this apparently, and beckoned him out of the room. She talked with him gently until he recovered and was okay to go back in again. There had been no subsequent reference to the problem between himself and Tessa, or anyone else. He seemed to think it was significant but he had no idea why.

"In fact, that was another thing I remember noticing about him; he really found it difficult to work out whether a personal issue was trivial or profound. I remember once we had a rather odd discussion as to whether he should serve Tessa with divorce papers because she had made a joke, over dinner, with a couple they knew well, on the subject of Marcus's dislike of Shakespeare!

"He was similarly knocked sideways when his cathedral mentor, a retired Anglican priest and writer, told him after five sessions of supervision over the course of a year that he would have to step down as his mentor because Marcus was, 'the most secular man he'd ever met'. Apparently, the old priest could not come to terms with the fact that in all their time together, Marcus had not mentioned the word 'God' once. Marcus found this implied criticism incomprehensible. By then, he had his exalted position in the cathedral management, still unpaid, and regarded himself as the cathedral's ambassador, I think. I wouldn't imagine that God was a big feature of the power politics which he was operating. The idea that the Almighty should have been allowed a toe in the water was obviously quite a shock to him, and made him fretful.

"That puzzlement of his always touched me to the core. Of course, I'd tell him about my confusions and shame ups in return. I'd describe the ways I'd failed disastrously or been told off, manipulated things, and of lies I'd told and truths I'd twisted, and he always seemed so interested. I suppose I felt as if he needed me as some sort of companion or guide to understand his own emotions and to get a grip on them. I found it very easy to help him because gradually, everything about him became more and more endearing to me.

"Perhaps he was just presenting me with edited highlights of his social confusion to lure me into a sense of importance to him! It was certainly very flattering to think that I might be able to help him not to compartmentalise and marginalise, as he phrased it. So, in answer to your question – finally! – yes, I think I was deeply flattered by him, but not so much by the compliments and the idealisations; far more by the completely mistaken idea that I could be of *use* to him, and encourage him to define his actions by relating them to his feelings, which he quite clearly could not do.

"In retrospect, I can see that the degree to which I was becoming internally focused on his identity and his thought processes was a form of trespassing, on my part. I might have acted as if I was detached from his internal reality, but the truth is that I had somehow let my own sense of Self get enmeshed in his. I thought that I sensed his confusion and loneliness, and I probably imagined he needed me alongside him inside his head to sort out the muddle. I justified it all in my own head by thinking of myself as some sort of private life coach, helping him to love his wife and family in a less declamatory, more internally integrated sort of way. How misguided of me to think I could make that sort of difference to him or to them! What arrogant stupidity!"

Alex sighed down at her bitten fingernails and twisted her wedding ring abstractedly.

Eventually, Jenny broke the silence.

"What about the whole 'Subject thing' you shared? I know that was very important to me when I was first getting to know Ricky. He seemed to possess a huge enthusiasm for all things artistically creative, and I was amazed by the energy with which he explored the art world, pulling me along in his wake. He had been involved with the arts all his life, from helping at summer festivals as a kid, through administrating a music school during his first marriage, to eventually gaining the professional qualifications he needed to work in the Arts promoting business. He was delighted to have done so! He had finally managed to make his apprenticeship steel working and HGV driving abilities redundant, as far as his own professional future was concerned.

"The joy he felt in being out of the orbit of manual labour and in the soft focus world of creative artistic enterprise was so infectious! Ricky really was a wonderful companion at any artistic event we attended. His enthusiasm was inspirational and utterly uplifting. It was wonderful to have someone else doing that for me, when I was much more accustomed to being the one to enthuse, doing the daily job of relentlessly encouraging schoolchildren's art work. Maybe you felt the same about teaching English, Alex? And then along came charismatic Marcus who lived and breathed the whole literary scene in his work and reputation."

Alex nodded, grateful for the observation, and continued to expand on the theme.

"Yes, but that's a funny thing, you know. Marcus didn't often quote his beloved Victorians, although he plainly knew everything there is to know about them. It was almost as if he identified with them as people, rather than felt inspired by their writing, though that may be unfair. He occasionally referred to them as, 'My fucked up, white male Victorians', especially Bailey, of course, who had stopped writing poetry by his thirties and then, after his conversion, wrote endless tortured diaries of complex theological philosophy. Marcus must be one of the few scholars who has read every word of those journals; he is *the* Bailey expert, I think.

"As far as I know, Bailey's immortal fame rests mostly on that early poetry, not on his elaborate metaphysics, but Marcus is an assiduous scholar with unbelievable reading stamina. He probably knew that if he cornered the market on Bailey's prose writing, no one else would ever have the endurance to rival him. I don't think he was moved by what you might call more accessible literary texts which addressed human relationships in some way or other. I remember him saying once that he didn't enjoy drama at all, and generally felt totally indifferent to Shakespeare's work. Kind of funny, isn't it? An English professor who doesn't like Shakespeare! No wonder Tessa found it amusing! I told one of Dan's brothers about it once, and he remarked, 'That'd be equivalent to a celebrated courtesan actually disliking sex!'

They both chuckled at this. There was a pause before Jenny spoke again.

"So why did we both repeat bad choices in men? We've got to get to the bottom of it, Alex, haven't we? Fundamentally, they were all our choices so we must bear the responsibility for them. At some level we can both read people. There must always have been warnings that these men – not your Dan, of course – weren't safe to love, but yet we both made the mistake twice over. What does that say about us? Why do we choose to break ourselves against the rocks? Is it just a variant of self harm, like Sharon Carter? You know, she was in my tutor group; a few years back, remember? She was regularly cutting her arms to ribbons and I missed it for one whole year!"

"Ah, if we really understood why we had chosen relationship meltdown, dear Jenny, I suspect it wouldn't hurt us anymore. I read somewhere that pain is a signal of wrong thinking. Once we've thought it out correctly, there's no need for the psychological alarm bell of inner hurt."

"But it never hurt when we were first in love with them, did it? What happened to your ruddy alarm bells then, when we needed them?" Jenny glanced over towards Alex enquiringly as she changed down into fourth gear, adjusting to the slower speed of a lorry in front of them.

"I dunno," replied Alex, after a pause. "Maybe fear and excitement feel pretty nearly the same. Did we recognise the tingle and urgency, but misinterpret that fear as the Passionate Frisson of Luurrve?"

"That stuff about the difference between the insanity of falling in love, and keeping your psychological balance while you actually love someone, come what may? Is that what you're on about?" Jenny's tone was uncertain, and she was frowning slightly in an effort to keep track both of the traffic around her, quite heavy on this stretch of road, and of what was being said. Alex pondered on a reply to this query for several seconds before she spoke.

"Well, I don't think I was insanely in love, either with Liam or with Marcus, to start with. Oh, maybe I was, come to think of it, with Liam. Well, at sixteen, I suppose infatuation's inevitable! Probably the only balanced start of a partner relationship I've ever embarked upon was when I met Dan once I came to London in 1980, almost a year after Liam left me. There wasn't really a chance to lurch into head over heels stuff anyway, back then. I had just found myself a full time teaching job and had two small kids, and my heart was still broken, I suppose.

"I was about thirty – same age as Dan – and he, too, had been unexpectedly deserted by his partner. He had insisted on being the resident parent of little Bella, who was about the same age as Connor, rather than agree to his wife's suggestion that Bella spend half the week with him and the other half with her. He thought that arrangement would be very unsettling for a five year old, and Bella was more of a 'Daddy's girl' in any case. So there we were, both single parents and both 'once bitten, twice shy' about the opposite sex's trustworthiness, at that point.

"Certainly, what we had was a friendship for some time before there was any sort of romance between us, let alone marriage.

I liked Dan from the start, but my liking turned gradually into a sort of grass roots loving of him. It's difficult to explain, but it was a sort of profound familiarity, which I felt about him much earlier than he came to feel about me. It took him five years to come round to the idea of the lot of us making a family together. I think maybe it was the closeness of Bella to the boys which persuaded him, rather than any passionate urge to live with me. But once we joined forces, sold our London flats, moved to Hampshire and set up home together, we were happy. It just seemed to work without drama or conflict.

"It was all in total contrast to the 'tip into it' urgency of falling in love with Liam fifteen years before, or under the spell of Marcus twenty years later! God, imagine being so absolutely stupidly enthralled by a slick conjuror at the start of my fifth decade! It's utterly incomprehensible in a middle aged woman with a good marriage. First time round though, I suppose it was understandable to fall for Liam, given that I was a lonely sixteen year old, with romantic longings."

Jenny said nothing and Alex interpreted the silence as a deservedly harsh judgement being made against her. After all, Jenny's involvement with Ricky, in many ways parallel to hers with Marcus, had not threatened resident spouses on either side. She glanced out of the passenger window beside her, resigned to processing the familiar feeling of shame, located somewhere in the pit of her stomach. It was a few moments before she could turn towards Jenny again, and switch the conversational thread to Jenny's experience of young love.

"What about you, with Joe? I know you were extremely cautious when you were getting to know Ricky because I remember talking to you at school about it once. I couldn't understand why you were so on your guard with him, not just when you'd first met him but for ages, as if you always felt it was all too good to be true. Were you like that way back when you first met Joe? Weren't you abroad or something? Was that love at first sight?"

CHAPTER TWO

Joe and Jenny

"Well, I first met Joe when I was twenty, and I was working for an animal charity in North Africa. My job was to help out the couple who were in charge of it. One day, I was in a chemist's and two young men came in, and the chemist asked me to translate what they were saying into French. One of them had got a streaming cold and wanted some aspirin or something, and anyway, I bought it for them. As these two young men were English, I invited them back for a meal because that was what we did with anyone we met who was English out there, and back they came.

"So these two young men spent an evening with us at the charity base and one of them, the one who hadn't got the cold, was Joe. Now he was very good looking. He was nineteen, with dark hair, blue eyes, a beard…. Bearing in mind this was the late Sixties, he was very trendy, you know, with boots and jeans and an old sort of pink duster jacket and a guitar slung on his back and he looked like – Oh dear! – a typical Sixties hippie. Anyway, back they came for a meal. They got on terribly well with the couple but for some reason or other, what he said and his whole attitude irritated me beyond belief; I can't tell you! I can remember exactly how I felt when I first met him. Anyway, then they stayed for a couple of days or so, irritating me even more, but I just got on with my work. Then, off they went to Algiers and the parting words from the couple who ran the refuge involved stuff about being welcome back when they were returning this way, etc."

A few tiny spots of rain suddenly appeared on the windscreen but not enough for wipers. Both women glanced up at the sky in front of them, but it still looked benign, a smooth light grey. Jenny was quickly back into African heat and dust as she continued with the story.

"Well, a month later, I heard these boots on the dirt track outside and I thought, 'That sounds like that awful Joe Allen', and it *was* him, though he was on his own this time because they had been fleeced of their money when they were in Algiers. His friend had gone off somewhere else and Joe had decided to come back. So he'd returned and he got in touch with his parents, and his grandmother was going to send him some money for him to get back home.

"In the meantime, he was offered board and lodgings if he worked for the refuge, which he did. Well, I had a reasonable social life; my friends were the French teachers who were out in Africa, sort of teaching. It was like a V.S.O. thing; French university students could opt to do good works abroad rather than go into the army to do their national service. So there were about three or four of these young French teachers out there, and I would meet them in their local hotel for a drink, and we would go out and – you know – have fun."

"Bet they loved you, Jenny!"

Alex was imagining the impact of a youthful Jenny's English attractiveness on a small group of marooned French men.

"Oh, we had a good time, certainly, but nothing sexual at all. I was far too inhibited for any of that! Anyway, Joe gradually ingratiated himself more and more into the work and life and so on. One day I said, 'Well, if you've got nothing else to do, come along to the hotel tonight', knowing full well that he didn't have anything else to do. So he came along to the hotel but I was meeting up with my friends and I was well in with these very good-looking French men. ('Jean-Jacques', one was called. Very tall and blond, he was; I can picture him, too!)"

Both women snuffled briefly in shared amusement.

"Anyway, after that, Joe started being rather nice to me, and suddenly, my attitude towards him changed, and I became totally smitten! We went off for a weekend together and we went swimming in the sea and I remember we spent ages just staring into one another's eyes! I'd fallen desperately, passionately, madly in love with him. We spent a night in a hotel and I wouldn't sleep with him because I thought that was all he wanted to do, and he was very chaste – we were very chaste that night; slept in the same bed, but that was all. Shortly after that, he asked me to marry him! It came totally out of the blue and I thought, 'Well, if I say 'No', that's a bit definite; 'Yes' is a bit positive, but 'I don't know' sounds a bit silly. I'll say, 'Yes' and I can always change my mind later.' So I said, 'Yes'.

"A couple of days later, he went back to England which was absolutely heartbreaking. We started writing passionate letters to each other. He had left Africa in the July but I wasn't leaving until the end of August. My parents at the time lived in the North, his lived in London, and when I was at last due to go home, I wrote and told him exactly which flights and dates and so on that I was arriving in Heathrow. The idea was he would come and collect me and bring me back to his house before I went home to my parents, bearing in mind that I was still quite young – only twenty. Actually, I don't think my parents even knew I was coming home then because I was planning just to turn up. Anyway, I had nowhere else to go! So that was where I was heading."

Jenny accelerated as she negotiated the move onto the Basingstoke bypass, transferring smoothly back into fifth gear along an almost empty road ahead. It was a gear change Alex silently registered since she had never managed to overcome her resistance to making use of fifth gear herself. She glanced across at Jenny who, quite oblivious of the admiration, continued with the narrative.

"Well, I arrive at Heathrow airport and no Joe! So I sit there and wait and it was much smaller, Heathrow, you know, and I waited in the Arrivals and I waited and waited. He lived actually not that far from Heathrow. So then I thought he'd obviously decided not to come and meet me. I sat there stunned for a while, and then it occurred to me that I'd go and stay with an uncle that I had in London – my sister's godfather. I knew where they lived and I was just about to go when all of a sudden, Joe tore in, rushed up to me and that was that!"

"From heartbreak to elation! Oh, Jenny, I can just imagine it! Weren't you furious with him?"

"Well, no, I couldn't be; not when I heard the explanation. Apparently, he'd only just walked into the house and found my letter on the mat. As he had arrived, his mother had also just got back in (she drove) and he'd said, 'I've just got to go!' He'd leapt into her car and sped to Heathrow. So it literally was sort of – if he'd been another few minutes longer, I'd have gone. I wouldn't have got in touch with him again and I don't think he knew where I lived. Oh yes! He *did* know, actually, because he had taken the train up north and made his way to my house while I was still abroad, to introduce himself to my parents! That had thrown them, as you can imagine, into a complete and utter quandary.

"I don't know why I'd ever previously endorsed the idea that Joe might be okay to do that, because I would have known perfectly well that my father would take an instant dislike to him, which he did. Joe was a Sixties hippie, after all, and my father, being my father, was not in the slightest bit impressed with what I was impressed with. And to have this young man turn up and say, 'I'm marrying your daughter' was intolerable. Dad was beside himself!

"Anyway once we're united at the airport, I then go back to Joe's house with him and we spend a couple of days there. After that, I make for home, still desperately in love and desperately missing this man, and wearing a ring on my engagement finger. It was a ring I had bought in North Africa (I still have it somewhere) for – like – five pence, it cost. So there I am back at home in Derbyshire with no job or anything – my poor parents! Then I just decide I'm going to go back down to London again, to live with Joe.

"My parents had been so pleased when I'd started at Art College the previous year, but within two terms, I'd suddenly thrown that up to go abroad, and now it must have looked as if I was completely off the rails.

"Oh dear! This is bringing back such painfully embarrassing moments because I mean, what about *his* parents? They lived in a three bedroom, semi detached house at the back end of Heathrow Airport. Imagine having this girl from a totally different background ringing up and saying, 'I'm going to come and stay with you!' What a nightmare for them! Joe's brother had said, 'Well, she's not having *my* bed!' because he thought that I came from Africa, and was an

African. So nothing racist there!

"Then, somehow or other, I go down and live with Joe and his parents and his grandmother. I have the front room and I get a temporary job. By now, we're having surreptitious sex. Every evening, Joe comes in and says goodnight to me and the last thing I imagine is that everybody knows, but of course everybody must have known because by this time we were banging away like nobody's business. (He had seduced me in the front room one day when his parents weren't there.) God, I feel embarrassed just thinking about it now!"

Glancing across at Jenny's profile, Alex smiled and nodded in acknowledgement of the enduring power of personal humiliation. Her gaze returned to the road ahead and the sky above and beyond it. Some darker clouds were now moving across the sky in watery wedges.

"Anyhow, we were still engaged; Joe used to introduce me as his fiancée, and at the time there were an awful lot of Sixties hippies living together and we were part of that crew. But we were the one couple who had declared undying love to each other and were going to get married. So we did! We went off to a Registry Office in Brentwood, and I got married in my grandmother's old fur coat with a minidress underneath, and my hair long and bleached blonde, and my eyes all made up big and black, like a panda. All our friends were there but nobody else – didn't tell my parents or anything like that – we just went and got married.

"I mean, I got a photographer. So I've got these photographs which say 'Proof' all over them because we never paid for them. We went to a pub afterwards and the manager came over with a bottle of champagne and we drank that......."

A weird image of a wedding photo appeared momentarily in Alex's mind, with the word 'PROOF' stamped right across it in huge red capitals, obliterating the features of the happy couple. The picture lingered with her while Jenny carried on talking.

"Oh, we'd told Joe's parents about getting married, and I think they had thought there was nothing they could do about it. So they had said okay, but after the wedding we had to go and live somewhere else. I'm sure they were fed up with all the bonking in the front room by this time! Mind you, it hadn't been all that long. We had got together in his house at the end of September and we were married on January 6th, 1967. I suppose I must have gone home to my parents at Christmas. God, how embarrassing!

"Anyway, we had found this flat in Teddington. It was the first floor of a terraced house which had been owned by an old couple, but she had died. The poor old husband had moved downstairs and he was letting out his top floor. There was a kitchen; there was a sort of a funny dining room; there was a bedroom, and the bathroom was downstairs in the kitchen – you know, there was a bath in the kitchen with a cover on it, and I had to tell the old man when I was going to have a bath, and lock the kitchen and the back door, and have my bath downstairs. Oh dear! They were funny times!

"We had decided we wanted to travel abroad and we spent our time planning it all out. We wanted to go to India to see the Maharishi. I was involved with all Joe's friends who were based in Richmond and Twickenham and Eel Pie Island, and oh! the Rolling Stones and all of that."

"My God, Jenny, you were so trendy! If I'd have met you then I'd have been in total awe of you; wouldn't have dared to say a word to you! Eel Pie Island! The Rolling Stones!"

"Oh yes! We certainly thought we were where it was all happening! We were out just about every night. I was working as a temp for IBM as some sort of an assistant in a lab, and Joe was working as a grave digger and also in a pet shop. We were spending our time planning our trip. Jobs and money were quite easy to get hold of at that time, remember? So we were saving quite a lot. Look – Greenham Common!"

Jenny nodded towards a road sign they were approaching, then alongside and swiftly leaving behind.

"That brings back memories, too; earnest days of trying to save the world from the arms race and nuclear disaster. Anyway, back to London! Are you still with me, Alex?"

"Riveted!"

"Well, I was desperately in love with Joe and it was just a wonderful Sixties type life style. There was lots of cannabis, although, to be honest, I didn't really like it and neither did Joe; Joe didn't smoke, you see, and I didn't smoke tobacco. So I used to just have a little pot pipe, but I pretended an awful lot, I think, that I was getting high. It seemed to me, though, that all our friends were genuinely high as kites! Anyway, it was a lovely time. We then saved enough money to go abroad. We were going to make our way down to South Africa where his godmother was. Joe had all these wonderful plans about what he was going to do and how he was going to do it, and we did our hitch hiking around the world and had lots of adventures, which are far too long to tell you now.

"There was one point when we were walking in Libya, trying to get down to Egypt and the Sudan which we did, but we were making our way along the coast. We had fallen out – there had been some big argument – and he had begun to irritate me again as he had in North Africa, and I just thought, 'I can't live with this man! I just can't live with him!' And I thought, 'I'm going to have to leave him and fly back home from Egypt.' He'd walked off, but there was nowhere for me to go because behind me was the road which just ran along the coast. I had to turn to follow him as the airport was ahead of him, and that meant I had to go that way, too. And we carried on walking in that direction, and then gradually my temper improved and I suppose we must have drawn back level again, and talked it through.

"But I do remember thinking to myself at that point, 'I'm stronger than he is!' I'd thought that he was a steadfast sort of person, but I realised that, in fact, I was a much stronger character than he was. That was a significant point, I think, in our relationship. And I decided that I could accept him for what he was. I could live with that. I said to myself, 'He makes me laugh, he's very good looking, he obviously cares for me, the sex is great, I have a good time with him, it's exciting, it's interesting: the pros outweigh the cons.' And therefore I thought that I'd be married for life.

"And then, of course, five months later, I found myself pregnant with Julie, and the rest, as they say, is history. We'd been away for about year, and when we came back, we came with absolutely nothing apart from four months' worth of a baby. Soon after that, my father reconciled himself to the marriage, dear man; it must have been very hard for him, but he did it. My mother's mother died and my mother gave me some money, and my aunt provided money too, and we set up the business. So that was it, really. That's how I met Joe.

"So what red flags did I miss there, d'you think? Why did he eventually throw out all our shared past so easily and move on without any lingering doubts or regrets, when once we had had it so good? How could I have spotted back then that I was on a hiding to nothing?"

"Oh, it isn't fair to ask yourself to spot that sort of thing at that age, Jenny! Surely we are just overcome that a man seems to be in love with us! At least, that's how *I* felt at that age. I wasn't going to start looking a miracle gift horse in the mouth."

"But I don't think I understood it any better once Joe left; and I was thirty by then. The 'why' of it all haunted me; still does, to this day. I was suicidal for ages, and then I suppose I began to pull through to survival mode. The kids saved me, actually. I had to pull it together for them."

"And me the same, after Liam left — Paddy was so young. I suppose both you and I must have been on some sort of maternal autopilot which even overrode heartbreak, though it was a close run thing. Yep, I think you're right, Jenny; the kids ensured our survival, but also made it inevitable that we wouldn't learn our lesson because we hadn't any energy left to look at what we needed to learn, back then. This time we do, of course. D'you think that's why it all seems even more painful this time round? Is it like a second kick on the shins? This time, perhaps, we're stuck with experiencing the total bone shake without distraction."

"And are we feeling it double bubble precisely because we didn't process it thoroughly enough, back then?" added Jenny. "Is that why it seems so mercilessly awful this time?"

"Well, if that's part of the explanation, we're certainly trying to do the processing to exhaustion this time round!" Alex chuckled. "You know what I'm like these days — the remorseless researcher, endlessly sifting through what I hope is the relevant literature, trying to find the key to it all in one easy sentence which will magically make us right in the head again, and free from the whole torment bit, once and for all."

"I'm glad you're locked into that process, actually. I couldn't wade through it, and it's probably necessary that one of us does. One thing that occurred to me the other day; if we're saying that these four men all had the same sort of fucked up defence system, and you say it's linked with early mothering which went wrong – too invasive or neglectful or whatever – why wouldn't all the siblings in their families have the same problem? The same mum would surely inflict the same emotional handicap on all the kids in the household....... But before you answer that, Alex, are you okay about us calling on Matt for coffee? Once we reach the M4, we'll have to turn off at Junction 17, but his place is less than ten miles from there. We're doing fine time wise, but, you know, is it really all right with you?"

"Of course it is! I'm so intrigued to see your wayward son transformed into the family man in his home set up! And it adds another level to this journey, seeing Matt a father, that bit older than his own father was when he left your family, although Matt's kids are quite a bit younger than yours were then, aren't they? But it's all about us breaking the chain, isn't it? And believing that because we've tried to do things differently, the next generation won't repeat the same mistakes? That's all we can ever hope to have done."

Alex paused, noticing that Jenny was indicating a turn off at the upcoming exit. She thought of her own driving anxieties, when such changes of direction needed to be made on fast roads. Jenny's directional adjustments, in contrast, appeared effortless.

"You seem to know this route so well, Jenny; no need for my crap navigation skills, thank goodness."

"Oh, I do this stage of the journey quite often, visiting Matt. This part is all very familiar to me but it'll be different when we get into darkest Wales."

There was a pause while Jenny was overtaken by a huge car transporter, and Alex resisted her nervous habit of clutching briefly at the front of her seat belt. She already knew that Jenny was both a confident and competent driver, and that such nervousness was misplaced. Once the car had smoothly acquired its steady speed on the selected route, Alex allowed herself to consider Jenny's enquiry, but kept silent as she did so, wanting to be sure that her friend really was prepared to be plunged, yet again, into her own obsessively investigative world. She gazed out at a distant stretch of pale gold land curving away on the horizon, half registering its beauty as her mind drifted back into exposition mode.

'The Development of a Secure Sense of Self

Thank you for your kind encouragement as I move into my second lecture, aware as ever that I am speaking from a layperson's perspective on matters of mental health which I have urgently and superficially researched while my audience's expertise is, by way of contrast, measured and long established. My only claim to speak publicly on such matters is that I have spent several of the last few years trying to regain a kind of mental equilibrium for myself, and it is in your field of knowledge that I eventually found the essential information I sought. I want to start with a brief overview of three key factors which help to shape our earliest sense of identity; a little trio of nouns which sit comfortably within common parlance and superficial understanding – nature, nurture and fate. I would like now to reflect briefly on the part each of these elements may have to play in one arena alone; that of the developing infant's sense of Self. However, I would like to take them in a different order, starting with fate.

"Fate may play a part in the infant's psychological development of identity over the first three years of life. The process of pregnancy and birth itself is rarely totally predictable, and things can go traumatically wrong through a combination of unlucky circumstances, rather than a failure in nurturing provision or an organic malfunction within the mother or infant's internal systems. Again, in the immediate aftermath of birth, circumstances may prevent the successful bonding between mother and infant, despite the mother's best intentions to nurture, and her healthy physical state after delivery of a baby with full potential to thrive.

A disastrous curtailment of the caregiver's supportive availability or some other external event(s) may subsequently cause a lasting distortion or stunting of her child's emerging sense of Self, especially if the unfortunate experience happens within the infant's first three years. Illness, accident or devastating catastrophe in the family and beyond it can have a huge impact on the circumstances affecting one child's development, while brothers' and sisters' experience of the same event may be very different.

Fate, luck, chance, fortune – whatever word we use to describe this unpredictable element which we cannot control – has become an unfashionable concept in some highly developed societies, since many would prefer to believe they are not subject to any negative form of it. It seems more rational to identify any significant problem emerging in earliest child rearing as an error in duty of care or a malfunction within the natural processes, rather than to concede there may be no responsible agent at fault, no inborn impediment to a successful outcome but rather, a profoundly unfortunate set of factors which affected the psychological health of the infant during a crucial developmental stage.

There are those who would argue that calamities like war zones, floods, hurricanes, earthquakes, fire, destructive states of mind, along with other devastating circumstances which can radically disrupt the support systems provided for the infant, are never just matters of fate; they could always have been prevented or alleviated, and are therefore attributable to a failure in nurture and/or nature, but not to bad luck. They may well be right. However, in a review of factors which influence a developing infant's emerging sense of identity, it would, I feel, be remiss to omit any consideration of the unknowable.

I now turn my attention to consider nature, which may very well have a vital impact on an infant's ability to develop a firm sense of Self. We have just glanced at some disasters within the natural world which may devastate a family's capacity to ensure physical and psychological well being for its young. There may, of course, be organic, constitutional or genetic defects at work within caregiver and/or infant which are also grouped under the term 'nature'. We may also speculate about aspects of the infant's temperament being inherited, and here we might cite, for example, the level of activity at which the child intuitively operates, ranging from very passive and relaxed to extremely excitable and curious. It is possible that a predisposition towards passivity, for example, in the infant may eventually have an undue impact on his/her emerging sense of Self if those who care for the baby are not naturally proactive in their alert attunement to the infant's emotional needs.

Lastly in this overview, I want to turn to the impact of nurture. We all started off as helpless infants, dependent on our primary caregiver, who was probably a mother or mother figure. Survival depends on a two way process between caregiver and infant, and a key ingredient for that survival is attachment. That word has two meanings at birth – the physical attachment to the cord, breast and/or the teat of the bottle, and the inner feeling of attachment which flows both ways between caregiver and infant.

Long before birth, a baby's development of physical and emotional stamina is profoundly affected if the connection between mother and infant is not fully functional, physically and psychologically, both via the umbilical cord and through the chemistry within the womb, responding to the stress levels within the host body. An all encompassing, attuned process of supply is equally vital subsequently, during the first months after birth. This potential experience of bonding comes under the heading of nurture, but the instinct to seek this profound attachment bond is hard wired into us, in the very nature of our being, to ensure the survival of our genes.

During early childhood, a wider provision of nurturing influences comes into play for many children. The support systems among relatives, friends and within community groups can vary considerably for each child of a family, and the degree of nurture available to each individual sibling may therefore differ to a marked degree. The caregiver's experience of nurturing within her/his own family of origin may have a considerable impact on the kind of care each young child receives, albeit unconsciously. Here, there may be particular factors such as the child's gender, birth order and/or level of attractiveness which spark off unidentified yet significant responses in one or other of the closest caregivers. Sometimes, this triggering may even result in the infant receiving a mode of attention particular to a parent's projections, created within a family of origin operating two or three decades previously.

A parent may be convinced that she provides the same loving support for each of her children, but long buried responses to how she herself was once treated among siblings may surface once she has children of her own. Birth order among the siblings may be a relevant element in the implementation of nurturing for each child, although exactly what this impact might be is unpredictable, since some caregivers improve their parenting skills as their family increases in number, while others use up most of their nurturing energy on their first born. Gender factors may be relevant too; some caregivers are profoundly affected by whether they are building a relationship with a son or a daughter, with a tendency to be more indulgent towards a child of the opposite sex. It becomes clear that siblings who are brought up in the same environment by the same caregivers may develop very differently, for all sorts of reasons.

So as I leave the topic of fate, nature and nurture, I suspect I have, at the very least, conveyed to you some of the complexities which have daunted me when investigating their possible impact on the early emergence of a sense of Self.

It is suggested that young babies have a sense of physical Self from at least the second month of life, if not before. As a baby plays with her toes, her sense of Self is working in two ways: acting, by making her fingers touch her toes, and feeling, by enjoying the sensation. By the age of eighteen months, fortunate infants develop secure attachment patterns which mean that they will be able to reflect a healthy sense of Self in relationship to their major caregivers. However, American studies suggest that in the U.S., over 30% of infants do not develop in this way, but instead develop an attachment style which is insecure in one of three ways.

Infant insecurity of attachment can be demonstrated by (a) avoiding a caregiver who has been absent for a brief period in a strange situation and has then returned, by (b) alternating between clinging to and resisting such a caregiver, or by (c) disorientated responses which have no pattern of consistency. Whatever style of insecure attachment has developed by the age of eighteen months will have a bearing upon subsequent adult styles of relating, although positive adjustment is possible through targeted intervention at any point in early or later life.

Research carried out in the 1990s has located an area of the right brain which may be considered the major neurobiological location for development of the Self. Between the newborn stage and a period around 18 and 24 months of age, the child's brain will grow two and a half times its size at birth. At this critical time, the primary caregiver, most likely to be the mother, may facilitate the development of the child's neural pathways as effectively as a supportive environment allows. If she does so, the unimpaired child will be able to become an active co creator in the development of a secure Self, through a myriad of intimate face and body language interchanges, as well as by shared tonal responses.

There are many other modes of self expression which will become available, to a greater or lesser extent, during the key developmental phases of childhood and beyond it. The more fortunate among us, the securely attached, are in a strong position to carry on discovering new ways to experience and communicate the Self in relation to the world round about us, whatever the challenges of our changing circumstances, throughout our whole lives.

A secure sense of Self is not something the infant is born with, but instead, it is something which s/he may be given the opportunity to develop. As I have already indicated during yesterday's lecture, this must surely be the best way to ensure the successful replication of our genes down through the next generations, given the need for adaptability and flexibility for each developing human being, in the context of his/her particular family and social groups.

By the age of three years, a child may have acquired this healthy sense of Self if s/he can recognise that the 'I' of one experience is related to the 'I' of another, even over a gap of time. Another feature of a secure sense of Self is the ability to identify how one has adapted to a particular interaction or event, and to feel empowered by this inner fine tuning. The securely attached young child will be able to call on some appropriate inner self soothing techniques if that adapting process has initially proved *inadequate, and significant discomfort has been experienced as a result.*

It will be thanks to the caregivers' validation and support, and through their provision of well matched environmental opportunities, that the three year old child may discover how s/he can achieve a growing sense of capability and confidence.

We can recognise the three year old whose attachment style is secure and whose sense of Self is grounded in success at mastering real interactions, rather than having to defend the Self constantly against damaging emotional states. Such a child can experience deep feelings, negative and positive, and is not afraid to be spontaneous. The self realised child knows what s/he wants, can express this and can defend these desires if challenged to do so. S/he is capable of some persistence in achieving an objective or maintaining a relationship, even if obstacles arise along the way. If there is a need to postpone or abandon a desired objective, the child is able to learn how to switch focus and, in due course, to come to terms with an acceptable substitute.

Part of the capacity to endure and commit comes from the developing realisation that s/he can use her Self concept to create enterprisingly different patterns of interaction, should the situation require them. Such a child does not live in fear of either engulfment or abandonment because s/he has not been made unduly anxious by caregivers who have over controlled or, at the opposite extreme, neglected the little one. The child has learnt to seek help as and when it is needed, and also to cope independently when self reliance is a valid alternative. These behaviours reflect a secure attachment style which will form the basis for all future .... '

"We're just approaching Matt's now!"

The words broke into Alex's internal presentation unexpectedly, and she instantly flicked her attention back onto what she could see through the front windscreen. She registered that they must indeed be nearing Matt's house, since the road they were now on was narrowing, and Jenny's driving style gave the impression of total familiarity with each twist and turn. Alex closed her eyes briefly, seeking to connect the content of her musings with the topic of Jenny's children.

"Well, both Julie and Matt seem pretty well adjusted adults to me, Jenny," she commented, hoping to link in with Jenny's as yet unanswered question about consistent mothering skills. "They've both got good careers and stable relationships and they seem to love their own kids. It was you who gave them that core stability and saw them through to replicate it in their chosen families later on. What an achievement! It must have been very hard on you with no financial support and being left on your own with them when they were so young. Were they nine and seven at the time?

"No, nine and eight. But it was just as tough for you, Alex, with Connor, four, and little Paddy just born."

"Ah, but you had two devastated kids on your hands while with mine, only one of them was heartbroken. Paddy didn't really lose anything he had ever experienced. Connor was certainly heart scalded when his dad disappeared.

"But I had an idea, back then, that children are most damagingly affected, in terms of self esteem, by a fracture in their relationship with the opposite sex parent, which meant I was relieved both my kids were boys, in the situation I was in. And there's the extra advantage that I had already trained as a teacher and was able to be earning a teacher's salary within a year of Paddy's birth. Eventually, too, I even got some child maintenance contributions from Liam. So I wasn't struggling financially the way you were. No wonder you considered suicide! I don't know how you made it, Jenny; I really don't."

"Well, I was very lucky to have really good friends and neighbours who saw me through. I don't think I would have survived without them. And Joe did eventually visit the kids every so often and took them out and so on. But he was very besotted with his new love – Molly: all of nineteen and a model, don't you know. I think being a father wasn't high on his list of priorities any more, by that time. From the kids' point of view, it might all have been quite a blessing in the long run, but it was a disastrous loss for them in the short term because he had been a great dad with them, as young 'uns. He left a huge gap in their lives initially, and it was one which I felt terrible about because I hadn't been able to keep their father resident, so to speak. Obsessive guilt again, eh?"

Jenny grinned briefly as they turned into a yet narrower road. Alex shifted her position in the passenger seat slightly, in preparation for arrival, and sighed in response.

"If only we'd known then what we know now, you wouldn't have considered topping yourself and I would have realised I'd been given an opportunity through being abandoned, rather than a tragedy. It took me ages to understand that some people actually thought I was lucky, at thirty, to have two kids who were healthy and full of beans, even without a resident husband. It just seemed a disaster to me, and I had no idea that I could give them a life as good as the one I had lost for them. Like you, I berated myself that I hadn't been able to keep their dad loving me and therefore living with us. I know that feeling of obsessive guilt so well!

"But at least I think I got one thing right. I always told Connor right from the start that his dad had got mixed up about giving the ladies he loved special hugs. I explained that Daddy thought he had to stop hugging me because the new lady's hugs seemed extra special to him, but that he still loved Connor just as much as ever. And that it was no one's fault, etc, etc. I had read somewhere that kids often blame themselves for a split between their parents. So I really tried to hammer that point home. Oh, is this it, Jenny?"

They were drawing up outside one of several older, semi-detached houses fronting onto the pavement. The attractiveness of its Cotswold stone suggested to Alex that it must be old; Victorian, perhaps? But the façade looked immaculate, the small shrubbery alongside the exterior wall beautifully ordered. She remembered Jenny's stories about Matt's aimless years as a teenager and young adult, and felt a moment's astonishment that he had, within a dozen years, acquired such a distinguished property. Jenny, however, seemed less dazzled by her son's social standing, clicking her tongue about the 'gas guzzling Four by Four' which stood large and proud in its shiny black splendour, close up against the garage door.

"I mustn't say anything, Alex – I mustn't. Kick me if I look as if I'm going to...." Jenny was now rummaging around under the back of the driver's seat for her handbag. "It's not my business what car he drives – he has his own life now – but oh, the planet, the planet!" She shuddered slightly as she straightened up again and closed her car door.

Alex smiled uncertainly, allowing Jenny to step in front of her across the gravel patch and over the threshold. From there, she knocked in a quick fire rhythm of raps on the interior glass door. Matt had presumably been awaiting their arrival, as both the front doors had already been left open in anticipatory welcome. It was a matter of seconds before he approached the inner one to usher them forward into the room. Mother and son embraced with brief warmth and he turned to shake Alex's hand. He was all smiles – tall, handsome, urbane.

"You remember Alex, don't you, Matt?"

"Well, yes, I think so, but it's years ago, isn't it? In my blossoming period?"

All three of them chuckled as they entered the sitting room, decorated in bright shades of buttercup and cream, and illuminated by the huge sliding glass doors at the far side of the room.

"Oh, isn't this lovely!" breathed Alex, taking it all in, and then gazing out into a long stretch of garden with open fields as a backdrop.

"Well, it's all very tidy, Matt," commented his mother dryly. "Where are the kids? It's awfully quiet!"

"Oh, Alison had to take them to some fancy dress party this morning. She's hoping she might catch you before you have to leave, but it only started at half past ten. I suppose it's unlikely she'll get a chance to pop back herself before you move on. They're just down the road – sight for sore eyes the three of them were, Alison walking off with her rather odd assembled regalia of princess and pirate......and the kids were in costume as well!"

Again, they chuckled. For all his lightness of touch, however, the coffee that Matt proceeded to make was meticulously prepared, smelt wonderful, and was served in stylish cream mugs on a glass table remarkably free from children's finger smears. By then, both women were comfortable on sofa and armchair, having toured the garden, admired all the downstairs rooms, separately visited the blue tiled bathroom and together exclaimed over the children's artwork which was on display all over the kitchen walls and cabinets.

Alex was deeply impressed by the combination of uncluttered elegance and child friendliness. The garden reflected the same skilful alliance: the beautifully constructed two storey wooden playhouse, the netted fruit and vegetable area, the well-kept lawn, tidy chicken coup, neat flower beds and three flourishing apple trees. One of these had a sturdy swing hanging from its lowest branch, which bordered the low wall right at the end of the garden.

Alex wondered how on earth the young couple had created and maintained such an ideal environment, given that they both worked and that their children, at four and two, were probably at their most demanding. She reflected that it might be no surprise, really, remembering that Jenny herself lived in similarly accomplished surroundings which demonstrated both practical and artistic talent in every aspect of house and garden. How people achieved this had always been a complete mystery to Alex.

She tuned back into the conversation between Matt and his mother which had moved from the little girl's considerable artistic enthusiasm and her younger brother's shyness to the potential danger of Matt's latest domestic project to keep bees.

"Oh, Matt! You can't have bees in a garden that size; not with two young children!"

"Why on earth not, Mother? There's no danger if the hives are efficiently managed. I'm going to do the whole thing properly, you know. There's a beekeeping course starting locally next month and I'm signed up for it already."

"Oh no! You're really serious about this! What on earth does Alison say about it?"

"Well, she was a bit dubious about it at first, but now she's as keen as I am."

He sipped his coffee and reached absently for a third biscuit.

"Let's face it, Mother, you'd absolutely love to keep bees yourself, given half a chance. You're just jealous."

Jenny laughed in reluctant agreement.

"Well, yes, I would, but at least I'd only be putting myself at risk if I did. Oh dear! How have I failed to imbue my children with a sense of parental caution and responsibility? Was I over cautious myself? Or too bohemian? One always gets it wrong somehow or other!"

"Well, what is this reckless journey you're embarked on now? You've been very mysterious about it. Why are you going to Wales, anyway, for just one night? I'm very curious about it all. Come on, spill the beans!"

"It's a sort of quest, I suppose. We'll tell you all about it in due course."

Matt suddenly turned to Alex.

"Can you elucidate? Are you being led astray by my wild and reckless mother?"

"Oh, goodness no!" laughed Alex. "Rather the reverse. I fear I'm a dangerous random element in your mum's life. She's the one in the driving seat who is handling the journey, coordinating all factors, map reading and driving simultaneously because I'm so useless. I never understand maps and their relationship to roads. I only remember routes by whether I've actually travelled along them before, and who with, and what we were talking about at the time. It's not a very reliable method, I'm afraid."

"Sounds a bit like Alison's filing system," commented Matt.

"How d'you mean?" Jenny tilted her head inquiringly towards Matt.

"Well, I was looking for something Dad had sent me some while ago; some stuff about another money spinning idea he had, car leasing; the usual sort of garbage. I hadn't even skim read it, and he was coming to stay the weekend. I rummaged around and then asked Alison if she knew where it was. She said she'd filed it. Well, I didn't bother to get it then and there, and when I remembered later, Alison wasn't around. So I went to the filing cabinet upstairs and naturally, I looked under 'C' for cars. No luck. So I waited until she got back and asked her. She seemed surprised that I'd had any trouble. It was obvious to her that it was filed under 'D'. Is it obvious to you?"

Both women looked at him blankly and shook their heads.

"Well, it was under 'D' for Dad. All stuff related to either her dad or mine is filed under 'D'. Didn't matter what it was about — if it had a direct link in her mind with either of our fathers, it belonged under

'D'. If Stan had sent her a recipe for making sloe gin, it wouldn't be filed under 'S' for Sloes or 'R' for Recipes, it'd be under 'D' because her dad had sent it. She said it worked fine for her."

"Yes, I get the idea," said Alex, with a grin. "I think I'd probably do it that way, supposing I had a filing system at all."

"So *did* your dad come to stay?" asked Jenny.

Alex, glancing across at her, saw that her friend's expression was benign, but there was a slight edge to her voice.

"Oh yes! This was a couple of months ago, now. It was the first time he'd ever given us advance notice, and actually stayed the whole weekend. Before that, he has hardly ever visited, and if he did, it was only because he was passing through, and usually unannounced. But, in all fairness, I do remember he had been adamant about coming down for a morning before the wedding. He must have felt it was important to meet Alison in advance of the big day!"

Jenny shook her head, tutting in mock despair.

"Oh yes! Who could forget him at your wedding?" she remarked dolefully. "He was on his very best behaviour at first, wasn't he? Charming to one and all! But then he began to lose it a bit, and a sort of pompous edge crept in, as he warmed up and got into his stories…"

Jenny winced slightly, remembering how she had felt to see Joe on that occasion, all too aware that she was on tenterhooks lest he somehow ruined this special day for the family. She paused before adding,

"But funnily enough, he caught himself somehow, and piped down after a while."

"Well, that was only because I managed to corner him, and have a few quiet instructive words," commented Matt airily.

"You instructed him?" his mother echoed in puzzlement.

"Yes, I've learnt that's what you've got to do with Dad. You just lay it out for him how to behave, if it actually matters to you for some reason. He is really quite amenable to the guidance; he can't read social cues by himself, you see. A wedding party is really confusing for him because he can't work out what he's supposed to do or be, but he has a nasty suspicion that the whole occasion is not focused around him. If he doesn't know what's expected of him, anarchy reigns, as we know to our cost, Mother."

"But didn't he resent your trying to control him? He was fairly well oiled and getting into performance gear. I'm surprised he didn't take offence."

"Oh no! No more than you would do if you needed to stop and ask directions on your journey. Dad doesn't even know that it's unusual to feel lost in that way. He imagines everyone else is as much at sea emotionally as he is. Well, to be fair, he doesn't know about being at sea rather than on land. He hasn't got a concept of what it might mean to be on firm ground when interacting with people. Curiously, though, he's great with the kids."

"*Is* he?" Jenny was patently astonished.

"Well, again, he needed some guidance about little people at first, and again, I'm talking about explicit instructions like, 'Sarcasm doesn't really work with three year olds, Dad,' or 'You need to speak in smaller chunks of words to her,' .... that sort of thing. But when it comes to play, he's very intuitive. He was right down on all fours with both of them in no time. He seemed to be able to tune on to their wavelength, and bask in their surprise and delight. He was quite taken aback when there was talk of bedtime, almost as if he was going to be banished upstairs as well."

"Well, I never!" Jenny leant back in the armchair abruptly, as if knocked off balance by this information. "You must tell your sister this! She's very wary of letting your father anywhere near her two, especially Timmy, who's such a sensitive little soul."

"Oh, she knows! We've exchanged reactions and tactics. But she's never had Dad visit her, as far as I know, for more than an hour or two when he's been passing through. She's not as laid back about it all as I am; never was. A bit of nonchalance so often does the trick, don't you think? You just say how you want things with Dad, and then step back, and somehow, there you are! It all pans out okay."

Both women gazed at him in some consternation. There was a pause before Jenny glanced at her watch and then up towards her son.

"Well, Matt, I suppose we'd best be on the move again."

She moved forward to sweep up the mugs and then walked towards the kitchen, adding,

"So sorry to miss the others! Send them my love; but I'll be seeing you all in a fortnight anyway, won't I? Saturday morning, wasn't it?"

"That's right. Oh, I've put by a few eggs for you in the kitchen, Mother. Hang on a minute and I'll just find an egg box for them......"

Alex rose as Jenny and Matt stood in the kitchen, sorting out details of a forthcoming family gathering. She moved towards a sideboard where some framed photos of Matt's family were displayed, all smiles and liveliness. Alison's happy face snuggled up to her daughter's in blonde conspiracy of joy in one photo, and in another, Matt, on all fours, had Holly and George riding astride his back.

She surveyed the images, letting herself drift into passivity, since the agenda of departure was not hers but Jenny's. She liked it that way because she sometimes found the smooth formalities of departure in unfamiliar social settings awkward to handle.

And then Jenny moved alongside her, grasping her arm briefly, and they were thanking Matt together, saying their farewells and gathering handbags before emerging into the front area once more. As they sealed themselves back into the car, Matt waved them off and turned back into his porch just as the car reversed back onto the road, swinging round to face the direction from which they had come. Then they were off again, almost on the stroke of noon, and as she accelerated, Jenny glanced across at Alex with raised eyebrows and a surprised smile.

"Well, would you believe it?" she exclaimed, giggling slightly. "Never heard Matt chat like that before about his father. Talk about taking the initiative in damage limitation! Out of the mouths of babes and sucklings!"

"Amazing!" nodded Alex, smiling in agreement. "Here are we, apparently heart and head scalded by Narcissist partners, while Matt can shrug off a Narcissist father like swotting a fly. He's made a wonderfully happy life for himself there, hasn't he? And he seems so relaxed and confident. It's as if he was quite immune from any harm his father could have done him."

"I'm not sure if I could claim he's undamaged, though," reflected Jenny cautiously. "Matt always has to appear affable in public, relaxed and unruffled, even when there's something seriously wrong. I think he learnt early on that hearts could be broken when adults said and did exactly what they chose for themselves. He seemed to pick up that his role was to be amusingly amiable under all circumstances. It works well for him in many ways, of course, but it still means he doesn't usually feel safe about expressing anything that genuinely worries him, and he is very uncomfortable if anyone else does."

"He must come across as very assured, though, when things look as if they might go wrong. He certainly appears to know how to handle his dad!" Alex commented. "But, in fairness, Joe doesn't seem to have engaged in the sort of character assassination which some fathers inflict on their first born sons; or if he did, it's all washed out very effectively."

"Well, from the time when Matt reached eight, Joe was hardly ever around," said Jenny. "Maybe – you know – that might be the most positive thing we ever did for our kids, as mothers; we lost them their fathers!"

They exchanged wry smiles at this as Jenny changed gear to take up position among other cars on a busier road, and they headed off for The West.

CHAPTER 3

Alex and Liam

"So, Alex – your turn. We'll carry on for about another hour, shall we, before we stop for a break. Is that okay by you? Run over for me the saga of how you and Liam got together."

Their speed was close to seventy miles an hour now, and the light traffic was moving steadily along in both the left and the middle lane, with only the occasional rapid overtaking of them by a car to their right. Alex readied herself for the narrative, casting her mind back to Ireland back in 1964.

"It's the tale of an Irish country bumpkin compared to yours, dear Jenny; real bogtrotter stuff. But quite a few similarities too, I suppose. I was also pretty young when I met Liam; it was back in our schooldays, sweet sixteen and all that, and, like you with Joe, it wasn't long before I was completely dazzled by him. But I wasn't doing something courageous in Africa! I was reluctantly playing a bit part in an earnest play being put on in the parochial hall, because a mate of my mum's was producing it. Come to think of it, the play was partly set in Africa, though! Liam had a role in it, too – he was playing a missionary, I think. Anyway, there was a row of us sitting on chairs against a wall during rehearsals one evening, and he passed down a packet of chewing gum. When it got to me – he didn't know me – he indicated that it should be offered to me, too.

"I remember being surprised and touched to be included in the gesture. The other three in the row were part of a group he knew, but I was an outsider. They were all mates from the local school friendship networks, but I'd been sent to boarding school in Dublin for two years and had only just come back to start my 'A' levels back in the North.

"I'd got used to thinking of myself as on the fringe of everything. So it never occurred to me that I might get a chance to interact, even marginally, with the Enniskillen teenage elite. Liam was very much the streetwise cool dude at the time, who had dated almost every pullable girl in town, according to the gossip. I had heard tell of him through my older brother's girlfriend, Liz. He was said to have wonderful amber eyes!

"Anyway, at these rehearsals, we began to talk now and again, and I felt very shy and awkward. I think I used to look up jokes in *The Reader's Digest*, equipping myself desperately with something witty to say, but he seemed to find me amusing whatever I said. I was amazed! One evening, we watched a dress rehearsal scene where neither of us was needed, and I remember we were in the dark hallway outside, actually holding hands behind our backs as we peeped through the gap in the side doors! I just couldn't believe that the fabulous Dyno Wight (his nickname was Dyno) would condescend to notice *me*, let alone want to go out with me, but he did!

"Within two weeks, when we were walking past the Roman Catholic cathedral, he suddenly proposed to me, and of course I agreed like a shot! We were inseparable from then on. I remember my mum was really quite put out about my lovesickness. For all my life up until then, I think I'd been rather a trial to her, following her around like a woeful little lamb, always wanting her attention. She was a great reader, and I well remember how she would look up, finger marking the place, when I, yet again, had something of urgent importance to tell her. She would wait patiently, with a kind smile, but then cast her eyes back down on the book to carry on where she had left off, as soon as possible.

"Two years at boarding school should have cured me, I suppose, but I think I returned even more soppily dependent on her than before, and now socially isolated from the teenage scene of Enniskillen where, before, at least I'd had good friends at the local girls' school I went to. Most accessible boys went to my dad's school and our house was actually part of the main school building. That meant that we didn't have neighbours and that made it difficult to be part of any local crowd. It didn't help that I had an English accent, wild, frizzy hair and breasts like fried eggs!

"So there was my mum, back to having her daughter moping around again until wham! Liam arrived on the scene, and my whole world abruptly revolved around him, instead of round her. Oh, my parents liked him okay. He was head of the Army cadet force at school, good at rowing and rugby, and he was aiming to get into Sandhurst. He was just the sort of dayboy my dad loved because he took all the best opportunities that a direct grant grammar school and boarding school combined could offer, and relished them. Liam saw no division between what dayboys or boarders might choose to do, and just took everything going.

"But anyway, I do remember my mum being very annoyed one time when I wouldn't go on a family boating trip one Sunday because I was going out with Liam. Any loss of time to be spent together seemed absolutely tragic to us then. Liam had a chance to go to England for a Royal School of Church Music training week sometime back then, and I remember my joy when he choose to duck out of it, rather than us be apart for a week; the music master was furious!

"Oh dear! How pathetic we must have seemed, and how ironic really, when it was all going to end in tears and heartbreak, as far as I was concerned. But back then, Liam seemed as crazily in love as I was. I regret to say, we were hard at it sexually within a couple of months, too. I never tried to fight him off at all, not like you with Joe at first, dear Jenny. My parents would have been horror struck if they'd have known. And I lived in terror of being found out or falling pregnant."

"Didn't you take precautions, then? I suppose this was before The Pill?"

Alex frowned with the effort of remembering.

"Uh, yes, I don't think The Pill became available until the late Sixties, or so. We thought the Withdrawal method was perfectly safe, and, for us, it turned out to be. But it was never very satisfactory, and I think maybe all that 'Get out quick' and fear of sudden discovery probably ruined our sex life permanently in the long run, even once all such precautions were unnecessary, either before and after we got married. Maybe we couldn't change the mind set, even if we changed the mode of performance. In fourteen years together, I later realised that I had never had an orgasm, but I was far too ignorant to work out that I was missing something out in the whole process. So it wasn't at all an issue between us."

"Quite surprising really – that even back as long ago as that, and in the wilds of Ireland, you were bonking away at sixteen!"

Alex glanced across at Jenny, whose eyes were on the road ahead, hands loosely placed on the upper curve of the steering wheel. For a moment, Alex felt another twist of shame in her stomach and wondered if Jenny disapproved. After all, Jenny had still been a virgin at nineteen, and had even held on to her virtue until she received a proposal. Alex sifted rapidly through a couple of defences in her mind before remarking,

"Well, I did presume that as I'd had sex with Liam, he must be the man I would marry. That was certainly a firm rule in my head, back then. I suppose I simply couldn't imagine ever wanting anyone else; he was The One! In hindsight, I think he might have felt like that about me for the first year or so, but once he went to Sandhurst and I started at university in Kent, unknown to me at the time, he had already been involved with the odd sexual dalliance here and there.

"I didn't meet any fanciable men during my student days but then, I wasn't looking. I wasn't cool (just an Irish bogtrotter, as I said!) and also, I was rarely in the social scene at weekends, anyway. I often went over to Camberley to stay in a B and B with Liam, or he might come to Canterbury and be sneaked in to stay with me at college. It was dangerous, that, because you could be sent down if you were found out. And, of course, the year I was in digs, there was no question of him staying in my room, which meant we always had to pay for guest house sex in Canterbury.

"It was a funny kind of time for me, really. I wore skinny tops and miniskirts and I was at one of the new universities, and longed to have straight hair that slid around in a shining clunk when you moved your head. And yet, there I was, the same awkward teenager, also turning up at Sandhurst church parades in earnest coat, hat and gloves, trying to look like an Army officer cadet's well brought up girlfriend!

"But much, much harder for Liam, of course. From council house Ulster dayboy to Royal Military Academy, Surrey; from pink shirt boutique wear in Enniskillen to kit from Gieves or Herbie Johnson's in London! It was a hell of a jump for him, and Sandhurst nearly broke him in the first term. I think the combination of deliberately gruelling routines and the need to jump a class level fast did him untold damage. He survived it and hung on in there, and even triumphed, I suppose, but he seemed to lose an essential – er – tenderness about him, somewhere along the line.

"That's an interesting little factor, Jenny, isn't it? Do you think it might be right to say that all four of our dear men had to switch class to get where they wanted to be? Might that be part of the Self disorder thing?"

"Well, Joe was certainly upwardly mobile in the same way that you say Liam was," remarked Jenny, with a nod. "They were both working class boys, I suppose, who wanted to live differently. And yet, you know, both of them have ended up without careers, with a series of broken partnerships behind them. So they never really made it into the social strata which they originally wanted for themselves, did they? Or was it that, having attained it, they felt compelled to reject it? Who knows!"

Jenny glanced at her rear view mirror before drawing out to overtake a truck, which seemed to speed up a little as she drew parallel. She was quiet for a few moments as she gradually drew beyond it and returned to the left hand lane, but then took up the thread of the conversation where she had left off.

"Perhaps, way back in the beginning, both of them used us as passports into another level of society. I suppose you and I both appeared to come from more privileged backgrounds than they did; our successful fathers and all that."

"That was part of Liam's magic for me, actually," smiled Alex. "It was so impressive to me that he had local downtown street cred; that he was *my* passport into Enniskillen and the local Ulster community who belonged there by right. I loved having high tea with his mum and dad and him in their kitchen, or talking with her about all the stuff of women's magazines and her knitting and her memories of her kids growing up. It all struck me then as a much warmer family set up somehow than my own, more intellectually-focused home life.

"His mum and I could yatter on for ages, and I really enjoyed her company. I suppose we also had a deep, unstated bond which was, of course, an utter devotion to her only son! That probably drew us together, heart wise. She certainly never appeared to be waiting for me to finish before she rapidly returned to her reading, the way my mum used to. Actually, didn't you say that you got on very well with Joe's mum? Seems that they were both devoted mothers, but yet apparently not at all resentful of their son's first serious girlfriend."

"Yes, Eileen was a 'salt of the earth' type! We kept in close touch for years after Joe and I broke up." Jenny's tone was affectionate, remembering her ex mother-in-law's consistent warmth and loyalty. She paused, waiting for Alex to resume her story.

"Yet, of course, by going to Sandhurst, Liam was on the way out of that apparently warm family and intimate community," Alex continued. "Perhaps it all felt far too restrictive and intrusive to him? There were certainly serious tensions in the family which I knew little about at the time.

"Anyway, I suppose I felt comfortable enough in the place he sought to be instead: in the anglicised world of English accents, tweedy people, golden Labradors, that sort of thing. I wasn't part of a set like that myself, but my parents were, because there was quite a little social circle of Anglo Irish folk who had country seats round about in Northern Ireland, as well as the London flat or the Cowes villa.

"Mum used to laugh at the phrase 'dirty diamonds', I remember, because some of the Fermanagh high lifers lived in glamorous discomfort back then. They had grand houses which were freezing and had mildewed curtains. They gave elaborate dinner parties where the hostess wore a thick black jersey over her long satin rig out, and the back of it was held together at the nape of her neck by a whopping diamond brooch, dulled with grime. 'Shabby chic', you'd call it now, I suppose, although that sounds phony. These people weren't putting it on. Their damp mansions really were bone chilling!

"It was all pretty eccentric, but somehow Mum and Dad were taken up into that circle. They were both Oxford academics but that wasn't their passport, I don't think; it was more that Mum was very good at networking, and Dad, as both headmaster and a clergyman, had a certain local status. But it was probably most of all because they were both good court jesters in a way; Mum always said they could sing for their supper! And maybe they were the token middle class locals. I remember something of the same in Army life. One wanted to pepper one's dinner parties with the occasional civilian couple; there was a sort of one upmanship, if you knew people beyond just the regiment or Army circles.

"Another factor was that the lake was a great social leveller. Upper and Lower Erne were a difficult pair of loughs; seven miles wide in places, thirty miles long in the lower part, and dotted with rock shoals and all manner of islands where all sorts of things could go wrong for sailors and cruisers alike. Dad was an obsessive sailor and also loved to bear people off in his chugging old cruiser, which frequently broke down. So that was another way he found himself on friendly terms with the aristocratic boat owners living near the lake shore. I think he loved becoming part of that world because he had come from a much less exalted home background himself, money and status wise, but Mum seemed pretty much at ease in that social milieu because her background had been more stable and much more privileged than his.

"Anyway, I'm losing the thread .... where was I? Oh yes! Liam going to Sandhurst that January. I was heartbroken, of course, to be separated from him, with two terms to wait until I went to university at Canterbury which, of course, I chose because of being handy to see Liam at weekends. (London or Reading would have been nearer, but I felt I couldn't cope with London, and Reading wanted Latin 'A' level which I didn't have.) Well, once he finished at Sandhurst, he was posted to Catterick.

"So, of course, my very first teaching job, which I managed to start the Monday after I'd done my finals, was at a little prep school in Yorkshire, only nine miles from the camp. It was a lovely job, actually! I had classes of twelve little boys in herringbone suits, and watched lots of very courteous Saturday cricket, and it left me plenty of time to do the newly required teacher training qualification by correspondence. And within a year, Liam and I got officially engaged.

"We duly found ourselves smiling out from a posed photo of us in the local Enniskillen paper, with me dolled up in a string of Mum's pearls! And then, the formal, appropriate wedding with pipers playing, and a guest list which largely consisted of my parents' social circle. Actually, though, it was all a bit muted because only a few months before the wedding, my brother Bryan had been killed climbing Mont Blanc, and it was still pretty awful for us all, and especially for Liz, his widow. I felt sort of ashamed to have the chance to marry my childhood sweetheart and to guess at her pain to be there on her own. Guilt, guilt, dear Jenny! How we are all corroded with guilt!"

Both women glanced at each other and shook their heads slightly, in smiling resignation. Alex shrugged and then continued,

"So there we were, such a conventional couple, unlike you and Joe. And it all started well enough, I suppose. We were posted to Germany within a year and enjoyed that, and then back to Northern Ireland, and then to Germany again, and then to England where Connor was born – a Lancashire lad, he was, born in Chorley! And then it was back to Germany again.......And that's when Liam began to go off the rails.

"I was very sad about it but I suppose not entirely despairing, thinking it was early days, and he had time enough to settle into married life eventually. I chose to see his romantic straying, which appeared to consist of getting traumatic crushes on other women whom he would suddenly long to marry and then subsequently forget, as being the result of depression brought on by alcohol damage. It seemed to me that the marriage itself was sound because I loved him so very much and every time we moved, I tried hard to get everything working at home the way he wanted it.

"To me, the cause of his lapses had to be alcohol consumption, though of course looking back now, I can see that his drinking was only a symptom. He had gradually developed the habit of heavy drinking during his Sandhurst days. His father had been a bit of a drinker too, although war injuries had severely limited his tolerance for alcohol. Both of them smoked like chimneys. Many years later, I found out that Liam's sexual dalliances had started very early on during his time at Sandhurst, and therefore before his drinking level had risen so dramatically.

"But at the time of his apparent romantic distractions, I probably feared most of all that we were both far too young to get married, and he had needed to sew a lot more wild oats first. Now I understand that what I'd thought of as his warm, cosy little family was actually just as dysfunctional as mine, if not more so, and that maybe it wasn't really a question of wild oats at all; it may have been more a question of shoring up his identity whenever the sexual opportunity arose.

"So there we are, dear Jenny! That brings us up to a parallel point in our romantic lives, doesn't it? Sorry to waffle on but it's interesting to see the similarities between our first hubbies .... d'you think?"

Alex looked across at Jenny with slight anxiety, aware that Jenny would have been very familiar with bits and pieces of her story anyway, and fearing it might have bored her to listen to a lengthy summary. As if to confirm her fears, Jenny glanced up from the map book on her knee and briskly remarked,

"Well, we're coming up to a view point pretty soon, I think. Shall we take the next exit and have a break for half an hour, eat our lunches and stretch our legs a bit? You did remember your lunch, Alex, didn't you?"

"Oh yes! I've got a huge pasta salad thing. There's plenty for both of us. It's from M. and S., no less!"

"Well, I've made my own sandwiches just the way I like 'em, and I've got plenty. We certainly won't starve. But I could do with a breather....."

"Of course! I forget how different it is for the poor driver, eyes on the road and negotiating fast flowing traffic while I prattle away, plucking me eyebrows, scrunching me toes or counting the age spots on the back of my hands!"

"Well, I prefer to drive than to be the passenger, actually. I quite enjoy driving."

"God, Jenny, you are amazing! I hate passing anything, and I am so likely to get lost on any unfamiliar journey because I have zilch sense of direction. D'you know, I had a career suitability test once in New Orleans. They never said you were bad at anything but they sort of suggested it by comparing you the national average. The feedback guy seemed a bit embarrassed when he got down to my lower scores. It came out that I am better than 3% of the American general population at Spatial Abilities. When I told Dan that, years later, he drew breath a bit, paused and then remarked that 4% of the American population is probably incarcerated!

"But it isn't only that I drive too slowly and might get lost. I am more afraid that I will lose myself. If I'm on a motorway with no familiar landmarks for long enough, I get scared that I will just keep going and forget who I am and where I am going and just fall off the edge of the world, d'you know?"

"No, I don't really," replied Jenny, with a slight shrug. "I think I'm quite at ease behind the wheel because I feel I'm in charge of all the elements inside the car, even if conditions outside are bad and there's a traffic snarl up. I just know I can handle things. I'm very used to long car drives on my own and they've never bothered me.

"But as a kid, you know, I was used to spending a lot of time on my own. I often wandered off quite a distance from home, just by myself. We were in the country and there was a big farm near us, and I just loved piggling round that farm and seeing what was going on there. Nobody seemed to mind, even if I climbed up into a tractor or stood near a horse's backside in a stable. Looking back on it, I suppose it wasn't a very safe playground for a kid on her own, but I loved it and I never came to any harm at all.

"My mum never seemed to worry. She herself had had a pretty harsh upbringing in the wilds of Canada, so I think she considered England very tame. I had a pony a bit later on, and I would ride for miles without anyone knowing where I was. I had tremendous freedom, really. I remember that I had already worked out my philosophy of how to deal with riding rules, way back then. If a time had been set for me to reappear back home and I knew I had already overshot it – say six o'clock in the evening – I would think to myself, 'Well, I may as well stay out an extra hour and enjoy it because the punishment for being two hours late probably won't be different from what I'll get if I'm only half an hour late.' It was quite a pragmatic strategy, really."

"How old would you have been then?"

"Oh, twelve or so, I think, when I first got my pony. And old Peggy Sue was as steady as they come. I think my mum just assumed

I'd be okay with her because of her ploddiness, and it was a fair assumption. One winter, I remember I rode her along some cart tracks right up into the hills, and suddenly the weather turned nasty, and we couldn't really make out where we were going. Everything was blinding white. Before long, she was up to her belly in snow, but she still ploughed on regardless, and we eventually found our way back home, no thanks to me. No one at home realised what had happened and I wasn't letting on because I didn't want my freedom curtailed. I suppose I was as sure as my mum was that Peggy Sue would always get me home, whatever happened."

"Where was this, Jenny?"

"The Peak District, Derbyshire – High Peak in Buxton, actually. Can be pretty bleak there. Mind you, Peggy Sue wasn't always ploddy. Once, I was riding her on a lovely spring afternoon in the Goyt valley. We were alongside the river when suddenly, I think the thrills of the new season hit her nostrils and she started cantering. I hung on for dear life but then she began bucking with joy and unseated me immediately. I came off and landed on my head, knocking myself out cold. When I came round, Peggy Sue was grazing beside me. I've no idea how long I'd been unconscious, but it felt like early evening by then.

"My head really hurt but there was no blood. So I stuck my riding hat back on, remounted and turned for home. Again, no one at home had been worried and I didn't say anything, but next day, I think I complained of a terrible headache which I claimed had suddenly come on during the night. As far as I remember, I even had the next few days off school! I must have come across as pretty frail somehow to my mum, who was a nurse and therefore usually insisted you went to school unless your temperature was well above 100. I suppose I must have been slightly concussed."

"Didn't all that put you off riding?"

"Oh not at all! I was just grateful that Peggy Sue hadn't wandered back home without me and given the game away. As it was, I was free to continue my solo riding just as I pleased, and that, of course, is exactly what I did. The Peaks are wonderful to explore, especially on horseback, because you see even more. I was really lucky to be brought up in that sort of countryside."

"I don't know why I wasn't more appreciative of Ireland's countryside," sighed Alex, shifting position slightly. "I think it was just a bit too forlorn somehow, and my dad was pretty casual about taking us kids down potholes and caves or up mountains, without any doubts about whether we'd ever get back again. He was always sure we would. But Mum would get anxious as night fell on a boggy mountain and all five of us were soaking wet, cold and hungry, and we couldn't find the place where we'd left the car. She never made a fuss, of course, but I think I picked up on her worry, and it didn't really help that my brothers always wanted to go deeper or higher or faster.

"So Mum and I were in the despised minority, as far as being 'sensible' was concerned. In fairness to my dad, we always *did* get home, none the worse for our jaunts, even if we were out on the lake on his broken down cruiser, being driven by howling winds into the nearest rock shoal. He always seemed to pluck victory out of the jaws of defeat, and would then claim we were never in any real danger anyway. He was probably right.

"It wasn't often the actual situation that frightened me so badly. It was if he got into a rage with the boat engine dying yet again or the car tyres being stuck in the mud or just running late to be home for Evensong. That really scared me because he looked to me as if he would explode. He never hit us or crashed the car or landed us in a real crisis, but his temper always felt like an imminent catastrophe to me. I don't think the boys or Mum were as scared of him as I was. They seemed more used to him, and perhaps had more faith in his ultimate control of himself than I did."

Alex sighed, wondering yet again if she had been a ridiculously over sensitive child. She continued in her familiar self reproachful tone, which made Jenny smile momentarily in recognition.

"I think that's why I'm such a physical coward in unfamiliar places; I just feel swamped by that old hyped up feeling of potential disaster and my own helplessness to avert it! And yet I'm sure that Dad wanted us to have memorable and exciting experiences which would feel good to look back on: shared with the family, achieved with effort and endurance, celebrated with chocolate which he doled out as 'emergency rations', and rounded off for me with a bouncing ride perched on his shoulders and feeling like a victorious team. It's so hard to get parenting right isn't it?

"Three kids in a family may all respond to the same enterprise completely differently: James, the eldest, learnt to hate Dad even more. That wasn't surprising, really, as Dad seemed to be an awful bully to him. Bryan, the middle one, learnt to love caving and climbing passionately, and the youngest, me, learnt to be a permanent coward. It just amazes me to think of you riding miles into the snow on your own, Jenny, without being afraid of the bleak solitude around you, but instead of that, learning the sort of resilience and independence which would stand you in good stead all your life."

"I may be quite self sufficient in my own company, but I am much more mistrustful of other people than you are, Alex, and I will rapidly withdraw into my shell if I feel threatened. So I think I can come over as distant or belligerent at times when really I'm feeling embarrassed or at a loss. You seem much more at ease with people than I am. I sometimes offend people without meaning to, because I can be a bit abrupt when I'm feeling ill at ease."

Alex was quiet for a moment, remembering how, in former days, she herself had misread Jenny's character as somewhat waspish. It had taken Alex some time to realise that they were gradually becoming friends, since she was particularly surprised by how Jenny seemed to sidestep farewells whenever they had spent any time together. A picture flashed in her mind of Jenny turning briskly on her heel and vanishing up her garden's little path as Alex had made her way towards her parked car beyond Jenny's gate. She had felt slightly hurt back then, but had eventually decided it was just Jenny's way.

"Well, I think I overcompensate all the time," Alex commented, stretching her legs into the well under the glove compartment. "I'm so afraid of being insensitive that somehow I overdo it, and probably come over as an intrusive cow half the time. I suppose I'm always trying to make up for the way I remember Dad intimidating people when he lost his temper. It used to horrify me to hear him shouting at James or a rowing cox, or at one of the caretakers.

"I remember one workman called Johnny, dressed in a boiler suit and carrying a bucket and mop, half running, half sliding alongside Dad who was striding down a long corridor of the school, black gown flapping, yelling down at him about something that had been badly done. I don't know what it was about, but I do remember Johnny's face, turned up, so pale and anxious, and he was stumbling along after Dad trying to drag the bucket of water and the mop along with it – so awful! To this day, I can't bear to hear even the slightest argument on the radio or television; I have to turn it off immediately.

"And yet Marsie, our cook and live in housekeeper, who started working at the school at the same time that Dad became headmaster, took no nonsense from him at all. She was swiftly promoted from being one of the linen room girls to being a sort of lieutenant for Mum, and she soon proved how capable she was at whatever she undertook. She must have been in her early 20's, and was a slip of a country girl from Derrylin, but she was very pretty and bright and feisty, and apparently Dad once asked Mum plaintively why the whole household ran according to Mary's rules, rather than his! (Her name was Mary, not Marsie; can't remember how or why we adapted it to our version but certainly, we children never called her 'Mary' and the adults never called her anything else.) She just had no fear of Dad at all and he was putty in her hands. He once quit a dinner party he and Mum were giving at the end of the main course to drive her to a special Mass in town. I remember Marsie was pleased about that afterwards because apparently he had told the assembled company, 'Please excuse me for a few minutes; I've just got to drop Mary down to Chapel…' She really liked it that she took priority over his exalted dinner guests!"

"But nice that he recognised that, too, Alex."

"Oh yes! He came across as a generous bear of a man who kept his word and believed fixedly in God, duty and loyalty. If it wasn't for his temper, he would have been truly impressive as a headmaster, anyway. But that was his fatal flaw, and once he was in a giant strop, he would become quite paranoid in his reproaches about being 'let down' by people. He seemed to feel particularly disappointed by James, which was inexplicable to some of the others who knew the family, and especially to Bryan and me. James was a really lovely older brother, kind and funny, and he'd come to comfort me, I remember, if I was ever crying in the night. He also had all the desirable qualities a parent might wish for in a son: looks, charm and the ability to succeed at almost everything he turned his hand to. But for some reason, he was never really valued by either of my parents when he was young.

"Maybe it came about through Dad missing a lot of James's earliest childhood because of being abroad in the war. Perhaps his father's eventual return meant that James abruptly lost a large slice of his mother's attention, such as it was; she wasn't actually the sort of mum who engaged with young children emotionally, preferring to use nannies and au pairs for that. Those two males may somehow have become rivals but it was hardly an even match! Mum would always have put her loyalty to Dad first. And Dad was pretty scary to an adult when he lost his temper, but to his own little son he must have been absolutely terrifying. I expect James became pretty defensive as a result.

"Bryan and I never copped it the way poor James did; I guess Dad expected less of his second and third child than of his first. He himself was the eldest of three and maybe that was part of the trouble. He never really learnt to be in full control of his temper, whoever he was with. The family legend had it that he and my grandmother were constantly at angry odds with one another, right from the start of his life, and the battle only ended with her death in her late eighties.

"Anyway, as kids, we all dreaded hearing Dad explode out of his study in a rage. He could calm down again in a relatively short time, and could apologise to Mum with real regret afterwards. I so wanted to love him as a child but actually, I think I was too scared of him to manage it, ever. Instead, I'm afraid I used to love it whenever he had gone off to conferences in England or anywhere else far away, because then everything was much more tranquil and I could have my mum more to myself.

"He was devoted to my mum, and he often really needed her guidance in terms of human relationships, especially as her background was part Northern Irish and she understood Ulster much better than he did. Her own mum had been American, a debutante from New Orleans, but her father was a good Belfast Presbyterian, who eventually returned to his home city when he retired; he'd been a doctor in the Indian Army Medical Corps. Mum was only five when her family left India for Ulster, which meant that really, Northern Ireland was her home country. As for Mum's take on Dad, she simply shaped her life round him, his faith and his career. Your folks were pretty devoted too, weren't they, Jenny?"

"Well, they were certainly a good team," replied Jenny thoughtfully. "Dad was high profile, of course, and his profession seemed to dominate our lives, in just the same way that your dad's did. He was The Voice of the Third Programme on radio, which meant he had to attend concerts all over the North, and sometimes in London, too. Obviously, it was essential for him to be punctual and in good health, throat wise. So how he was, and whether things were running according to plan were the dominant priorities in our household. It became equally important whether his hair was the correct length, and his shirts and handkerchiefs were properly ironed once he began to read The News on television. Oddly enough, though, his shirts had to be pale yellow, not white, on account of the glare from the lights.

"Anyway, my mum certainly ensured everything he needed was always ready exactly when it was required. I would have thought that it worked like that for the majority of couples back in the Fifties and Sixties. It was the accepted norm at the time, surely, that the man was the wage earner and the woman the homestead manager and child rearer? I know Mum would have liked to have bucked that trend because she had loved her nursing and even tried to return to it once I started primary school. But Dad was always very jealous and insecure, as far as she was concerned; I think he really disapproved of her going back to work. I used to say to her, I remember, things like, 'Why don't you do just what you want to do, Mummy?' but she'd just laugh and say, 'If I can't go back to work, I'll just have to have another baby!' Which, of course, she did!

"My father was a volatile man, like your dad. We would all creep around when he was in a bad mood, because it didn't do to get in the way of his wrath. He used to slap us hard if he lost his temper but he would never have hit Mum. There could be a very grim atmosphere around the house, but it didn't seem to shake Mum much; I think she knew that she was the stronger one of the two. She ran her empire very much her way, and there's no doubt that Dad really had very little personal access to his three daughters because that was her province, not his. So he was cornered out of any intimacy with us and never quite knew how to approach us, I think. Perhaps the frustration of that made him more likely to shout or slap."

"Would your mum ever have stepped in to protect any of you from a random, undeserved thwack from your father?" Alex was concerned about this childhood experience of injustice.

"Oh no! I don't remember her ever doing so. It wasn't as though he had lost control when he slapped one of us. We probably had run too noisily past his study or hit the window with a ball or something. Both my parents were products of very much harsher childhood regimes themselves, which meant that the odd undeserved wallop here and there didn't register on their Richter scale. It did on mine, though! I remember I often wished heartily for my father and elder sister to be dead; then I could have my mum to myself, though I was magnanimous enough to spare my younger sister from fantasy extermination, on account of the fact that she was rather sweet, and angelic by nature; still is!

"I think perhaps she was almost too good because Mum still found herself with time on her hands, even when Wanda was very little. My mother was the sort of person who always had to be busy. But she certainly found lots to do in her needlework and her charity work, and if she resented Dad's curtailment of her freedom, it was never apparent to us. She was very proud of him and what he had achieved, and she was consistently supportive of him, even if she didn't always see things as he did. It was a good marriage, in the culture of the times. You'd say the same about your parents, wouldn't you?"

Jenny glanced across at Alex, with a slight tilt of her head.

"Oh yes – they made better spouses, I think, than they did parents, but that was probably the culture of the times, as you say." Alex tried to swallow a sense of anger she felt about some of the parenting skills she had witnessed as a child, particularly between her father and his elder son. She continued to recall her own family's dynamics, struggling to match Jenny's non-judgmental tone.

"As a couple, my parents certainly had great fun together and I think they really brought out the best in each other. I don't think

Dad found it easy to relate closely to anyone else. Mum said it was because his own mother was a control freak who was totally self absorbed and incredibly argumentative. Maybe he was damaged by a Narcissist parent? D'you know, I'd never thought of my grandmother as a Narcissist, but of course she may well have been! She'd fit all the criteria perfectly."

"You don't think we just see it everywhere now?" asked Jenny. "Like when you're buying a certain make of car, you suddenly chalk 'em up all over the place, whereas before you'd never noticed them at all?"

"Well, if about one in fifteen people is seriously relationship dysfunctional, surely we are pretty likely to encounter it somewhere in each generation of the family, and also among the people who we'll get to know – or to know of – in a lifetime? It may not always be a rigid Narcissistic defence but all the disorders in the Cluster B group are shot through with narcissism anyway."

"Remind me what 'Cluster B' is again...." Jenny asked this from a position of genuine confusion, but she also knew how much Alex would enjoy giving her an answer.

"Well, Personality Disorders can be grouped into three categories, remember, according to whether they are the 'A' sort, which are usually about very odd behaviour and are therefore fairly easy to spot, the 'C' sort which are again pretty easy to identify because they involve behaviours like extreme anxiety and dependency, and the Cluster 'B's – my favourite!" Alex chuckled briefly at her own absurdity.

"Any of us, whenever we're cornered, may exhibit any number of defences from one or other of the clusters. But to my mind, the cluster 'B' defences are the most interesting because they are grouped together under the heading, 'emotional, of interactive impact'. So these are the ones which are going to deceive and bamboozle other people most. The Cluster 'B's are all about concealing underlying emotional mayhem, and putting on a false front, aiming to be in subversive control of significant others. After prolonged contact with someone who is far along a cluster B disorder, a person being targeted will probably get infected, somehow or other. That means the emotional mayhem spreads!

"Borderlines, Histrionics, Narcissists ..... they're just variations on a theme – all Disorders of the Self which will do in the head of the people in closest relationship with them. The only type in the group which probably won't gradually send their nearest and dearest bonkers is the one labelled 'Anti social' because he or she probably won't even try for a sustained relationship in the first place. But Anti socials are somewhat more likely to con you, exploit your trust, damage you financially or physically, or even, worst case scenario, dispose of you entirely! "

Jenny glanced across at Alex with a quick smile, registering the firmness of tone which indicated that her friend was fully in exposition mode. She offered up an appropriate question, knowing that Alex would scarcely pause before answering.

"What if two relationship disordered people get together? Do they end up doing each other's head in?"

"I don't think so. I think sometimes they can be in a sort of collusion of reciprocal supply, so long as they aren't operating competitively in exactly the same field. If one of them isn't willing to be of use to the other, they won't get intertwined anyway, since both of them will be seeking supply from the other in some way, and either one will back off if this isn't available.

"I suppose it would be better if the various highly dysfunctional people who can't really 'do' positive relationships always paired off because they would probably do less additional damage to one another than they would to a more functional partner. They can be content in the 'non relationship', I think, in a sort of unconscious collusion of stuckness. It's far less demanding and aggravating for them that way than coping with the complexity of bonding with a reasonably functioning person. It would be massively frustrating for them if their partner is gradually learning from experience and developing, to some extent at least, and therefore cannot really be controlled.

"A dominating man can be particularly irritated, to the point of towering rage and beyond it, by his 'functional' woman's apparently natural ability to express her feelings effectively, to form supportive networks and to connect openly with her friends, broadening her understanding in the process. A controlling woman, however, is likely to be luckier in her search for dominance since her targeted, 'functional' man is usually less likely than a female to be expansive about his own feelings and those of others, or to have close friendships which often involve analysis of relationships, and is consequently much easier to isolate. She can make short work of getting him stuck too, crushed into adopting her defensive systems."

"But aren't we all disordered to a greater or lesser extent?" enquired Jenny. "What you call a 'stuck defence system' is just a particular way any one of us might use to protect ourselves when we feel threatened. Isn't it perfectly normal to be abnormal?" Jenny chuckled at her own illogicality.

This question appealed to Alex even more than the previous one. She had spent a considerable time trying to work through her own muddle on this very point, and had only recently begun to clarify her own take on normality. She was just taking a breath to commence her answer when Jenny gesticulated towards a sign ahead on their left. "The rest area is coming up in a mile; shall we take that turn off?"

"Good thinking, Hawkeye!"

Alex considered expounding on normality but thought better of it.

CHAPTER 4

Breaking the Journey

Within a minute they were turning onto the slip road, and they were soon speculating about the best viewing spot to select alongside the grassy verge, their speed slowed down to a crawl. The rest area was surprisingly extensive, almost like a mini park. There was a superior sort of display stand, made of wood and steel, between two of the benches. It offered an engraved map, identifying landmarks in the spectacular vista spread out beneath them. They selected a parking spot near this sign, and Jenny turned off the engine.

Two boys were riding mountain bikes up the slope which marked the limit of available space but otherwise, the whole facility was empty of people. The sky still looked grey but in the far distance it seemed rather brighter, with a gleam of silver stretching along part of the horizon. The two women rummaged in their bags for their packed lunches and then pushed open their nearside car doors. Alex remained seated but Jenny sprang out to stretch her arms wide and throw her head back, circling her shoulders. She ducked down to address Alex in the far side seat.

"Shall we eat on one of the benches?"

"Yep – just coming!"

Once seated on the cold wooden slats of the bench, Alex placed her container of salad and her boxed drink alongside her, and gazed out at the landscape beyond them. Jenny sat to her right, with her carefully wrapped sandwiches on her knee. She was already drinking from her bottle of water and, having taken several gulps of it, she put it down again and sighed contentedly.

"That's better – I was really thirsty. Matt's coffee was dehydratingly good!"

"He's grown into a very handsome young man," commented Alex, taking up her sealed bowl and plucking ineffectively at the top edge of it. "Who'd have thought he'd get his life so beautifully organised, when you remember his extended period of being prone on your sofa, munching crisps? I've never forgotten that tale of your having to collect him from some party or other at an unearthly time at night and as you were berating him in the car, he stayed silent for a long time and then he turned to you and asked gently with a dear smile – what was it? – 'So you don't want to be my Mummy anymore?' I just love that story!"

"Oh yes! Matt could always turn the tables on me, however cross I was with him. But, you know, he never forgave me for forcing him to leave home. He still mentions it occasionally, and never as a joke. Yet I honestly believe that if I hadn't done that, he'd have stayed watching TV from the sofa for ever. He refers to it as 'the time Mum threw me out' as if he was an orphan in a storm."

"How old was he at the time?"

"23! Looking back on it, I suppose he was depressed and maybe, in retrospect, I can see I could have handled it a bit differently. But it worked! In the end, he went back to college, met Alison and, by hook or by crook, he got things together, found a good job, got married and became as materialistic as any other ambitious young bloke. But in his mind, that was despite my cruel abandonment of him, not because of it!"

"But he doesn't really still resent it, does he? Usually parents get forgiven for all their supposed sins once their children become parents themselves!"

"Oh yes! He still festers about it all right, but he doesn't rub my nose in it so often now. Here, Alex, give me that! You seem to be having trouble."

Alex passed over the salad pack, and Jenny instantly pealed back the top, handing back the plastic bowl with a helpful "The plastic fork is fixed inside the lid." Alex nodded her thanks, giggling at her own incompetence. "I'd be much better at opening things if I didn't bite my fingernails," she remarked regretfully.

Jenny made no comment because she had a slight aversion to the habit, and always tried to avoid catching sight of stubby finger tips. She remembered that she had once helped Alex to make a clay slip cast of her own hand, in order to demonstrate the technique. The resulting model of Alex's left hand was successful enough, but the clay fingers reached out from a broad wedge above the wrist and the total effect was of a rather ugly chunkiness.

They munched their respective lunches and gazed down at the view. The air felt cooler than in Hampshire, but they were both grateful for the fresh breeze.

"That could only be England," Alex commented between mouthfuls, nodding down towards the land below. Jenny followed her gaze before replying,

"Actually, it's probably Wales as well; those blue grey hills on the horizon."

"No, but I mean it couldn't be a different country, like Ireland. You know, a different landmass. You'd never get a view like this in Ireland."

"Why not?"

"It's too well composed, too organised and elegant. Ireland is so much scrubbier. I have to say, I love the civilisation of England. You're rarely far from a good pub or a well-kept public toilet or just houses and lights and – well – people."

"But surely that's what's wonderful about Ireland? Its wildness?"

"I know it is, but somehow, I had too much of its wildness. You could feel quite forlorn and bleak there, in a way that I've never felt in England. Probably comes from too many narrow squeaks on those family adventures. And there was one time Dad and Bryan and a few others had to take part in a long drawn out cave rescue. I think it took a whole day and night to get the stretcher down the pothole, reach the injured man and negotiate him back through the underground passages, strapped on the stretcher, without doing the poor guy any further damage. They got him out in the end but he was badly concussed. He had weeks in hospital and I think he had double vision for a long time afterwards. I seem to remember that he didn't make a full recovery."

"Dangerous hobby, potholing, wherever you choose to do it," commented Jenny, biting into her second sandwich.

"Yes, I know, but somehow, that sort of thing stuck in my mind. I began to link the beauty and remoteness of Fermanagh with danger and death. I know people die in the Lake District and that there must be dodgy cliffs and caves in Cornwall and Devon but somehow there feels to me more of a rescue infrastructure here. It all feels less risky, and perhaps that's because more people seem to explore the wilder places here than they do in Ireland. So in England you'll round a scary cliff edge and suddenly come across a hotdog van or a bouncy castle or something."

"You'll be saying that you prefer crowded beaches with funfairs and casinos next!"

"No, beaches are different somehow. I really like them being empty and far from civilisation. Daft really, isn't? After all, you might need rescuing from an undertow or a shark or something but that never seems to worry me if there's sand and sun, though, of course, you didn't often have sun in Ireland. That's another thing! The weather in the south of England is so benign. It doesn't often blow a gale or rain for days on end. I just love that! Oh dear! I really have become a Soft Southerner, haven't I?"

Alex slurped on her straw, tipping her boxed drink to extract the juice at the bottom.

"Well I never thought I'd end up living in Hampshire," commented Jenny, with a sigh. "It seems so predictably tame to me, too, after Derbyshire, but that was another time, another life, and I suppose I've packed it away in my mind. I've had to do that because otherwise, I'd yearn for the wildness of it all too much. I think I regarded the Great Outdoors as my companion when I was small. I never felt uneasy about being in danger or anything. Maybe that's because riding Peggy Sue meant we were a team together. I think I felt safer outdoors than in, really. My older sister and I really didn't get on, and somehow I often felt out of step in the family. It's classic middle child syndrome, I expect!"

"Terrifying how everything seems to root back in the past," sighed Alex. "Puts such huge responsibility on you as a parent, when you realise how critical those early years are."

"Yes," nodded Jenny. "How does that Jesuit motto go? 'Give me a child until he is seven and I will give you the man' .... something like that. The Catholic Church certainly grasped how critical childhood was, in terms of influence. Unfortunately, a few of the priesthood have grasped the opportunity only too passionately, in horribly perverted ways."

"Not just the Catholic priesthood, though. Child abuse by elders crops up in lots of other cults and religions, too. I don't think even the ol' milk and water Church of England has been immune from the odd scandal about molested choirboys." Alex was keen to put her father's religious domain in the frame as well.

"Yes, but I think it's bound to occur more frequently when young men have to renounce their sexual desires to enter the priesthood," reflected Jenny. "I'm not sure, but I think most other variations on the Christian faith don't stipulate celibacy. I would imagine that a religious man with a network of close friends and/or one steady partner and maybe kids of his own would be far less likely to be sexually frustrated and stressed out by the denial of his physical urges. I expect someone somewhere has researched this subject very thoroughly!"

"But it might be the other way round, mightn't it?" suggested Alex. "Maybe the kind of young man who chooses to go down the celibate priesthood route is unconsciously attracted to the rituals and discipline of the brotherhood community because he actually craves that restricted all male environment. And what he craves may be the opposite of intimate heterosexual relationships, which he might imagine be too threatening. Instead, he may eventually be given an opportunity to be in a controlling position over his congregation, especially over women, gate keepers to their children.

"He could be someone more driven to influence and dominate than to connect. Perhaps if a rogue Catholic priest abuses a child, it may reflect his perverted sense of power and control over the most vulnerable members of his flock. He believes he is God's representative on earth, after all, and he would consider that he has a right to appropriate any lamb exactly how he pleases, but best to choose the ones least able to object. I think it's sometimes a matter of the corruptive influence of power, more than repressed sexual desires."

"You mean that sometimes these men were dysfunctional, even potential exploiters, before ever they became Catholic priests?"

"A select few of them, yes," nodded Alex. "And only dysfunctional in the arena which you might label 'mutual loving relationships'. Intimacy and sustained mutual support were just too dangerous for them to contemplate. If you look at the core beliefs set out for the Catholic church, it's interesting that the only woman who gets venerated has pulled off a double act which is impossible for any other female – that of being both virgin *and* a mother! Very useful for male solidarity if the brotherhood promotes an ideal which ensures failure for every other member of the Virgin Mary's sex! In that failure, all women are deemed to be falling short of an ideal.

"And somewhere back in the first few centuries after Christ died, a group of powerful Christian men decided *that* was the best spin to promote. And it is still apparently unthinkable to the Vatican men at the top that there should be women priests, for example, or that women should be able to make their own choices about avoiding pregnancy. So surely if a young man chooses to dedicate his life to this set of beliefs, he must, at some level, be at ease with the idea of men having a higher religious calling than women, and the need to avoid being distracted by them? It's a comforting ideology for men who want a good reason to avoid intimacy with women, isn't it? But it also serves to promote male bonding, I would have thought; this idea of exclusive male authority reaching up to the dizzy heights of infallibility.

"Come to think of it, isn't it Cardinal Newman who was buried with his long term male companion, and now he's on the way to being declared to be a saint? He seems to have been a dedicated sort of priest, a theologian who wasn't just full of abstract rhetoric. I think he said something like, 'the love of our private friends is the only preparation for the love of all men'. Apparently, his closest friendships were with younger men who were sort of disciples to him, and he maintained a profound relationship with one of them, a fellow priest, for over thirty years."

"I'm confused, Alex. Are you claiming that the Catholic Priesthood promotes male bonding at the expense of connection with women? I guess we would both agree that being an oddball isn't about whether you're gay or straight, it's about never wanting an intimate balanced relationship with a responsive adult of either gender."

"Er – I'm not quite sure *what* I'm saying! Perhaps I mean that if we constantly seek to avoid any sort of mutual close relationship, something may have gone wrong for us somewhere in our family of origin, that's all. But how convenient that there is an institution which tells us (if we're men, of course), 'We will only accept you into the hallowed ranks of God's representatives on earth if you renounce intimate human relationships which involve personal attachment either to women or to men.'"

"But you've just said that Cardinal Newman is being made a saint, and he was buried with his beloved male friend," Jenny pointed out. "So doesn't that mean that this present Pope must now be recognising that it's okay for Newman to have been committed to that close relationship and also to be a Cardinal?"

"Ah but I think I read that they attempted to exhume the old boy from the grave he shared with his friend, and pop him in somewhere else in solitary splendour. In other words, the Catholic hierarchy wanted to erase Newman's most significant relationship, but celebrate his piety by canonising him. Now that seems a really bizarre plan to me; to desecrate the grave arrangements which Newman himself specifically requested, and to justify this violation in the cause of celebrating Newman's sanctity.

"By all means plonk him somewhere more sparkly if they want, but shift his mate's bones along with him. Why not? The other guy was a priest too and probably a very good type. It seems to have been a friendship based on intellectual and spiritual closeness, but I remember reading that Newman said that his friend's death felt to him as dreadful a loss as mourning your husband or wife. So it sounds like there was an intense emotional closeness as well.

"As far as I remember, though, the Catholic hierarchy didn't get their way in the end. The two friends weren't separated in death after all, since the waterlogged ground apparently swallowed up all the bones, and only a few pieces of the Cardinal's tassel were dug up."

Both women smiled, touched at the poignancy of this image. Alex shifted position slightly before pulling her attention back to her line of thought.

"I'm burbling on again, aren't I? Sorry! Um – I think the trouble comes when we try to control others for our own sense of empowerment. It's bound to be an abusive process in individual relationships and it is, in my opinion, just as much an abuse of power in institutions. It strikes me as daft for an institution to try and legislate how people should run their private relationships with mutually consenting adults. I think any such relationship which provides consistent, mutual and sensitive support, allowing both parties to flourish in their own spheres, is a wonderfully healthy achievement. It should be celebrated, surely, not mudded by prurient speculation or official embarrassment."

"Prurient?"

"Um – I'm not sure what it means, myself; certainly couldn't spell it! I think it means like a peeping Tom; having an unhealthy curiosity about the supposedly erotic elements of other people's lives. It would include sniffing the crutch of a girl's knickers, for example. Presumably the girl herself wouldn't find knickers she's been wearing a turn on, but a prurient person might."

Jenny breathed a half chuckle at this definition. "I always remember you saying in the staffroom once that just because you were an English teacher, it didn't mean you could spell. That really surprised me. I used to be so in awe of you, back then – well, Head of English – I thought you must be so intelligent!"

"You know better now," sighed Alex, with a wry grin.

"Yes, I know now you're just weird. But that's okay – I can hack weird!"

"The English always consider the Irish weird," replied Alex, smarting slightly. "I think they want to despise them as illiterate, but it's a bit hard when some Irish writers and poets have outdone their English rivals in brilliantly creative use of their common language. We're always uneasy, aren't we, with those people and events that have contradictory characteristics or effects: 'A terrible beauty' and all that. I think 'weird' is a shorthand way of saying we can't pigeonhole someone. Under that definition, I'd say you were weird too, Jenny!"

"So we're both odd–balls? Is it that which makes us targets of Narcissists, d'you think?" Jenny took another swig from her water bottle before continuing. "I would have thought a Narcissist would want a conventionally desirable partner – a sumptuous trophy woman – to accentuate his high social status to others. Why would zaniness attract them? They might get tainted by association!"

"I suspect it's simply that they don't recognise that we're odd–balls. They don't read social subtleties accurately because they are too busy trying to conceal their own edginess. I remember dear Marcus once telling me with considerable smugness that work colleagues of his were often exceedingly surprised when he rang them up on the day of their birth. He kept a record of all relevant birthdays, in order to be able to do this. He told me that the recipients of these birthday congratulations of his were often amazed to receive them, thanking him with bemused gratitude. He seemed to think it was evidence of the warmth of his friendships at work. But I suspect that for some of the colleagues, his phone call might have come as something of a shock. Ringing people on their actual birthday usually suggests a closeness which borders on family membership, doesn't it? But maybe I'm wrong about that. Perhaps they were delighted and touched. It just seemed a bit strange to me."

"Well, Ricky's reading of social cues could be very odd, too. I remember being with him once on a picnic, with Sandie, his daughter, and her friend, both aged thirteen at the time, and his oldest son, Alistair, and his girlfriend, who would have been eighteen or nineteen. The girlfriend's parents were with us as well. Ricky was larking around with the teenagers, playing some sort of rounders game, and getting rather over excited by the whole thing. Alistair and his girlfriend had had a bit too much beer and were beginning to show off a bit, using quite a bit of bad language.

"In no time at all, Ricky was outdoing the pair of them, both with his beer consumption, and with the most inappropriate profanities you can imagine, and this in front of his own daughter and her friend! The girlfriend's parents were horrified, and I didn't know where to put myself. In the end, I had to draw Ricky aside quietly and suggest he might want to be a bit more sensitive about his use of language. He toned it down a bit, but seemed unconvinced that it would have caused anyone a problem.

"And – the same sort of thing: I remember that we were taking Alistair back home to London on another occasion, and we drove by a building which Ricky identified, in passing, as a convent. He cheerfully pointed out, 'That's where you were for five months of your young life, Alistair!' It seemed by his half laugh in response that Alistair already knew about this, but I didn't, and later on that evening, I asked Ricky what he had meant. Ricky explained that he and his wife had a flat not far away from the convent when they were first trying to establish themselves in England. Once Alistair was born, they had found their new baby's crying very troublesome, and had given him to the nuns to look after.

"Eventually, both sets of parents back in Ireland had got wind of this, and her horrified parents had come over straight away to take baby Alistair out of the convent and back home with them. Ricky and Thalia followed not all that long afterwards, and settled back in Ireland again. They started up a music school of some kind, I think. She was a singing teacher and they went into partnership with some musician friend of hers, but they couldn't get it established. Anyway, they did take Alistair back before his first birthday. The odd thing is that Ricky was very nonchalant about telling me the story and apparently saw nothing unusual at all in what he and his wife had done. I was a bit dumbfounded at first, but you know how it is, Alex; you sort of talk yourself round to thinking it was quite normal, yourself."

"Yes, it's amazing how easily we came to absorb any shock waves they transmitted!" Alex agreed. "Marcus told me about some odd things he had said or done sometimes, and because he saw nothing strange about them, I came to accept that it might be perfectly reasonable to slap your troubled adult daughter across the face for being unappreciative, or to leap angrily out of the driving seat of your car which was ticking over at traffic lights after your wife, sitting beside you, had mildly objected to your driving panache.

"Generally, though, Marcus kept his impulsive gestures well under control. I think he may have had some awareness that he was actually in an extremely alert frame of mind, and that he needed to disguise this because others might find his defensiveness weird. He may even have some idea that so called normal people bimble along with an apparently random sequence of internal monologues playing in their heads. This bimbling is certainly *not* what is going on internally for any of us when we're in a state of shock or of extreme urgency.

"If we can relive the sort of no man's land we enter at crisis point, then I think we can experience for a moment how adrift the Narcissist feels most of the time. Marcus would sometimes ask me suddenly, 'What are you thinking?' I was always utterly enchanted when he did that! I thought I mattered so much to him that he even wanted to share my unprocessed internal chatter as it happened. Now I think he simply wanted to understand how an inner stream of consciousness operated."

"But surely anybody else's stream of consciousness would be pretty chaotic to another person? Think of Joyce's *Ulysses*. I'm totally stumped by Molly Bloom's internal monologue, and I've got it in print to pour over it in my own time, in detail. (Not that I would, of course.) Aren't we all foxed by one another's thought processes?"

"Well no, I don't think we are," replied Alex. "I think for most of us, our inner burbling works rather like Molly Bloom's self talk stuff; it meanders along with a sort of basic connectedness, despite the jumping around. I don't mean we think the same things as her, but the process of thinking – brain chatter – probably operates similarly for the majority of us. But I guess that people with stuck defence systems have trained themselves to be perpetually on guard against attack. So they are different from most of us who are chugging along quite nonchalantly in our own inner stream stuff. But our particular Narcissists chose to *act* as if that's what they're doing too, and appear to be laid back."

Alex was looking towards the distant horizon, chin tipped up. "It must be extremely difficult for them, actually. Like having to give a speech in a foreign language and trying to conceal you're not using your mother tongue. I suspect that their internal reality is always stressed, however relaxed they may appear outwardly. And along with that, I think they feel they are liable to be zapped out of existence at any moment, if their precarious construct of human interaction is somehow challenged. It's vital for them to be able to control the inner responses of those who are close enough to ask questions.

So I think a Narcissist operates from stress, fear, and a pathological need for control, as well as from anger and envy."

"Why the last two?" Jenny was glancing at her watch as she replaced the top on her bottle of water. "What are they angry about? What have they got to be jealous about? I just don't get it."

"I've wondered that," mused Alex. "All four of our men had looks, charm, charisma, talent, adoring mums and seemed set on a path to success, didn't they? As they got into their stride, they all made successful transitions from working to middle class lives, at a time when that was probably more of a challenge than it would be now, for our kids. On the whole, they weren't explosively angry men; indeed, Marcus prided himself on being Mr. Cool, and Ricky, you say, appeared deliciously at ease and full of sparkle in the spotlight.

"Yet from what I've read, Narcissists can only access the most raw, defensive emotions, not the socially learnt ones like empathy or regret. I think there are eight – what is it? – er – primary emotions. I can never list them all but it's anger, disgust, fear, anticipation, surprise, sadness; that sort of thing. I think if one was preparing to battle with an enemy, hyper vigilance would make most call on anger, disgust and fear, wouldn't it?"

Jenny considered this information for a moment before responding, "Surprise if the enemy ran away, and joy if that meant one could then raid the other's habitat. But you mentioned envy as being on the baseline. Surely that isn't a primary emotion? I can't imagine a Neanderthal man gazing enviously at another's bone necklace!"

"No, I don't get that, either. Yet apparently people with Narcissist Personality Disorder are driven by envy. I've read it in lots of different stuff. I would have thought one would have to learn to envy others; it seems a sort of social emotion to me, or rather, an anti social one. But perhaps envy is a combination of two primaries, like fear and anger working together? It might be – er - anger that Narcissists feel themselves to be somehow less functional than other people, and fear that this will emerge somehow. It's all about shame too, and deflecting their own vulnerability onto others. I dunno."

"What about sex?" asked Jenny unexpectedly.

"How d'you mean?"

"Well, what d'you think is the Narcissist take on sex?"

"Hmm. Difficult to generalise, isn't it? I haven't read much on the subject of sex, as far as relationship disorder is concerned. Assuming our four men fall within disorder somewhere, let's consider their attitudes to it. Sounds as if Joe and you had mastered blissful delights at an early age but, in retrospect, Liam and I weren't great at it. I remember I liked it okay, and was always up for it, hoping for closeness, but we certainly weren't adventurous. I don't know if he fared better with the one or two other women he'd already tried before we got married, although I do know that things must have really taken off after he met Helen in Nigeria. She would know a lot about bodies, one way or another, being a highly qualified nurse. She had worked abroad for some time, I think, and had had quite an exotic time in Singapore, before she had got married. I guess she knew a sight more about sensual delights than either Liam or I did, and that must have been electrifying for him! I managed to sneak a read of one of her letters to him which he had left unhidden by mistake, just before he left me. It sounded as if they were having quite a romp. I was obviously a very damp squib compared with her!"

"But sex with childhood sweethearts is always likely to be pretty fumbling and basic, isn't it? I'm asking about sex with – er- mature Narcissists, if that's not a contradiction in terms! What are they after, with sex?"

"Don't ask me, Jenny! You've had more good sex with admiring men in your life time than I could ever dream of! For Gawd's sake, you were having a passionate affair with a local doctor within five months of Joe's departure! I'm on the nursery slopes here and you're off piste!"

"But I'm not talking about numbers, Alex," Jenny grinned, half acknowledging Alex's admiration for her startling repertoire of conquests. "I'm asking what Ricky and Marcus – fridge set Narcissists rather than wobbly, just gelling ones – might have wanted out of sex? Why should they engage in it at all? Men lay themselves on the line with sex, performance wise; they can't fake an erection, after all. So why would a Narcissist allow himself to be open to that vulnerability, especially as he got older and the hydraulics might be faulty? And surely, also, if sex works, it encourages intimacy, and it appears that they're running away from that. What does sex supply for them, then, d'you think?"

"Good question! From what we've said before, neither Ricky nor Marcus were particularly driven by sex when they started up with us, were they?"

"Not at all! Ricky apparently had another woman in mind when we first met, and actually asked someone at work which of the two of us he should shack up with, once I came on the scene!" Jenny's tone was incredulous. "It was probably hard for him to weigh up the potential use of either of us to him, all by himself. I think he must have been considering a whole package of provision, rather than being driven by uncontrollable lust for my body!"

"And with me, Marcus seemed perfectly content with a romance without sex arrangement: you know, 'snatched kisses behind the water fountain' – adolescent sort of stuff – but nothing full on. In retrospect, when we first met, he must have felt less threatened by me than by most women because I was his unpaid employee, and I expect being the boss of a diffident woman who had offered to assist him in his professional role was a subconscious green light for him to make use of me in any way he liked. He was just toying with me, and had no real desire for intimacy at any level. I would once have said that the reason for that no sex pact between us was that both he and I wanted to be faithful to our spouses, but long after he dumped me, I learnt, through a casual conversation I overheard about him at Uplands, that he was sleeping with at least one woman – maybe more than one – when he was on fund raising tours abroad. (Maybe that was part of the fundraising effort!) I was surprised to learn that, but not exactly upset. After all, he was Tessa's husband, not mine, and I've never felt I owned a man sexually, or vice versa."

"But yet we both did end up in an intimate relationship with these men, didn't we?" insisted Jenny. "Ricky and I actually lived together for nigh on eight years. What did sex mean to them? Why bother with it? You've said Marcus spoke positively about regular marital sex with Tessa; he wasn't gagging for it with you, then. And Ricky – well, we had rollicking times okay, but I don't think it was anything other than an enjoyable lark to him. To be fair, though, he could sometimes be touchingly personal about me. He never failed to admire my bottom, which was exceedingly good for my morale! But he was keen on experimentation, I remember, and I was pretty accommodating, although less enthusiastic if it hurt.

"Towards the break up, there was a lot – a lot – more hurting. I even began to wonder if he intended that. It must have been at the same time as things were picking up with la belle Madeleine. Maybe he thought if all that bedroom stuff became rather unpleasant for me somehow, and he was off hand enough during our daily life together, I'd be the one to break it off with him, and he could go straight on to my replacement without hassle, or him having to own up to his lies. I do think Ricky was a coward – and Joe, too, come to think of it."

Jenny looked distressed at this memory, and drew breath before continuing. "I remember Ricky was away in Spain, allegedly looking at possible English teaching jobs there. I had resigned from the Girls' school two years previously, because we were going to go off together, we knew not where, and he was looking at possibilities. He had had a disastrous year in a new job in Ireland, and that meant we weren't going to establish a base there. Everything was up in the air back then, and I was worried because he seemed very jumpy, but I thought that was inevitable, given the enormous battering his professional pride had taken. He had believed the Dublin advertising job was a wonderful career move after the routine stability of the Arts Council role in Hampshire, but far from it! The whole thing had rapidly turned out badly for him, in every possible way.

"Anyway, I'd gone out to Ireland to be with him and then, after he had lost that job, I'd come back home for a while, doing supply teaching locally. Every so often, he'd return before going off for another job research trip here, or extra training of some sort or other there. Things were becoming tense between us, but I truly believed we could work it out, especially when we found what we wanted to do and a new location to live, a fresh start together, really. It was only a matter of time, I thought. We were in touch by phone and by email if he was away, and I was able to earn quite a bit by the supply work, so things looked okay-ish.

"And then, quite early one morning, I rang him up when he was in Spain and his voice sounded odd; he was obviously still in bed.

And I asked how things were, and he answered, and then I just burst out suddenly, 'There's someone in there with you, isn't there?' And there was this awful pause, and then he just said, 'Yes'. And it all fell into place, all the odd little actions and words and inconsistencies which had puzzled me here and there for so many months, but that I'd chosen to ignore. The only one that had consciously disturbed me – which seemed to be a warning somehow – was the fact that he hadn't been tender with me anymore, when we made love.

"So – um – I wonder if their apparent tenderness is just a way to keep the sex on tap, for as long as we're their main supplier? Is there no genuine personal affection or spontaneity in the whole process for them at all? It's all so horrible, isn't it? I suppose we have to accept it was only ever one way: what we felt about them." Jenny sighed deeply.

"Hmmm. Could it be that sex is for them just another form of control over their woman?" Alex was reluctantly considering an idea which was new to her. "They don't want intimacy, but they do want power over every aspect of their supplier, and her physical availability and loving responsiveness is part of the domain to be commandeered.

"I think Marcus eventually began to feel a need for greater power over me. He had lost the director post at Uplands suddenly within a little over a year of his appointment, and therefore I no longer worked for him. The reasons for this unexpected departure were hushed up to avoid adverse publicity for the project and a sullied reputation for Marcus himself. Apart from his anger and resentment about it, and his claim that his envious employers had sacked him because of the adulation he received on his tours abroad, Marcus gave nothing away.

"But you know how it is, Jenny; the various Indians within an organisation each know basic stuff about their Chiefs, and whisper about it with one another when going about their lowly routines. So Marcus's cheque to finance the entire clean up operation for Uplands' computer network was processed through my mate, Tracey. Even if the matter was kept under wraps, it must have been unbearable for Marcus, to find himself so humiliated. Perhaps he found a slight consolation in a new use for me, at that point. Maybe he felt he needed to establish himself as my boss in a completely different sort of location, far away from the scene of his private disgrace.

"I guess there were other reasons why he wanted surer ground to operate in. He probably felt threatened at times by our increasingly personal talks together, where I must sometimes have strayed near the source of his covert defensiveness against others. Certainly, it was about that time when he started trying to be more demanding with me physically, and I had a hard job fighting him off. If he ever feared there was something questionable about his psychological state, perhaps, by way of contrast, his management of the sexual arena would have felt much more assured to him.

"I wonder if having sex is the closest a Narcissist thinks he can get to a 'normal' connection with a woman. As long as all his erectile systems operate, the chances are, he might think, that he employs a honed technique which works at least as well on a woman as any other successful lover's approach. I expect, too, that sometimes he gets a kind of random sexual itch which just needs an instant gratifying scratch with his handiest supplier. Maybe that's unfair, though. It could be that there *is* a blissful moment for him, if it goes well, of genuine, undefended union with another human being. It might be his only way of achieving that profound connection, however briefly.

"What Marcus didn't have, however, was integration between his body and his mind. I learnt that once during a conversation we were having over a cup of coffee at his place. We were reflecting on men and women's insecurities about being attractive in the bedroom. I remember him gasping and going white as a sheet, when I made a positive comment about Dan's reliable operational efficiency. It was a casual remark, quite in tune with a familiar conversation we were having about gender attitudes. Marcus was analysing his love for Tessa and his frustration that she did not always seem to enjoy his company during a routine evening, even though she was always up for ardent sex. (We spent a lot of our time considering how he could make Tessa happier; it was a constant theme of his. I think he was unnerved about her devotion to the children and to her increasingly high powered job, feeling that he only came third in her priorities. I was certain that she had a profound devotion to him and their marriage, and I pointed this out whenever he was doubtful, but he still remained unsure of his central importance to her.)

"Anyway, I'd just made this passing remark about Dan's sexual fitness when Marcus seemed to sort of sway. He was standing near me in his kitchen at the time, I remember. When I asked him anxiously what was the matter, he said a white hot splurge of pain had shot through his body. I was very alarmed, thinking he must be ill. He sat down for a minute or two, and gradually the colour returned to his face. Eventually, he seemed to work out what had happened, and said he had been similarly shot through with pain a few times before in his life, in just the same sort of way. He suspected it was some sort of intense feeling. In this case, he suggested it might have been a sharp pang of jealousy but it had now dissipated completely. He dismissed it as a topic of any curiosity, but privately, I thought it was surely evidence of a sort of disconnectedness within himself.

"In our last year of meetings, what happened between Marcus and me was never about mutual passion; it was about trading vulnerabilities, physically or psychologically; a sort of quid pro quo, I suppose. Marcus assured me that sex with Tessa worked very regularly, with prolonged mutual enthusiasm, he said, and that as a couple, they were entirely unaffected by any aspect of his dealings with me. I believed him, and I suspect it was completely true!"

Alex was aware of using a sort of defensive word mist to shroud the detail of what she was saying. If Jenny was also aware of this, she appeared, by her impassive expression, to be disinclined to challenge the evasiveness, much to Alex's relief. With a nervous glance sideways, she moved herself rapidly onto safer ground. "I think maybe Marcus used the imagined responses of admiring women to shore up his constructed identity as an enormously sexy man. Dan is totally different, of course. His self fulfilment tended to focus on outdoor strenuous exercise, like training for the next marathon, or perfecting his kite surfing, which are lone pursuits, I suppose. Indoors, his delight is in the Voice, opera and all that, and those aren't joys he actually needs to share with anyone else. He certainly never sought female admiration or attention, the way Marcus did. He was the very opposite from a snatch and grab man! Tuning in to a connectedness between us was easier for me than for him, I think, and I certainly have never felt like a femme fatale to him. But we could get very close at times, especially when we weren't bowed down by work pressures. Affection and reliable performance were much more natural for us both than intense urgency, steamy sort of stuff.

"So I must admit, ... er ... I was amazed and flattered once Marcus had begun to ditch the Courtly Love idea, and seemed suddenly to find me incredibly sexually attractive, especially in that urgent kind of way. No other man in my life had ever responded to me like that! I presumed that it meant Marcus was by now too passionately in love with me to be able to restrain himself! I was honoured, I suppose, that he considered me desirable, but guilt and inhibition made it impossible for me to be swept away by him.

"I suppose the best occasions with Marcus for me were the couple of morning hours when he would open his mind and heart to me in his study about his writing and his academic world, and then we would walk and talk and go for a pub lunch and I'd feel that we'd been in a sort of spiritual connection, not fervent physical coupling which would obviously be fraught with potential pain to others. If we were playing 'The Writer and his Muse', he would celebrate my empathy for his work but then move on to say delicious things to me like 'I'm the only man who has ever really understood the Very Soul of You!' and I would accept that as wonderful, momentous truth. Spiritual connection, indeed! It was all nonsense, of course. I was under his spell and he would keep weaving it, consciously or not, for as long as I was of use to him.

"I think Tessa got annoyed, eventually, that even though he'd left his job, I was allegedly still doing research for him for his next book (so I was), and meeting him 'to report back'. Who could blame her! She had been bewildered by why he had lost the post at Uplands, and clearly no one was going to give her the real explanation. But at least the dismissal made it clear to her that Marcus and I had no need to be perpetuating working links between us. I'm sure she demanded that the arrangement ended, and it promptly did. I was devastated, and particularly shocked by his curt break off by email, but I believed he had done the right thing, for the sake of his marriage. I didn't know, back then, about any other woman in the background at the time, although I guessed that his dodgy use of the internet probably included some interactive sex sites. Perhaps he dumped me to put Tessa off the scent about the other ones! Who knows? I think I'm blithering here, Jenny!"

"Well, we can continue with blither in the car," smiled Jenny, as they rose from the bench and made for the public toilets. She cleared her throat, nodding briefly, but there was something in her face which suggested she was in need of a swift diversion from thoughts of the past. "But we must get back on the road now, if we want to make Much Wenlock by mid afternoon."

"This was a great place for a pit stop," said Alex, with a nod back towards the picnic area. "I hope it was enough of a break from driving. It's a long ol' slog for you while I sit with me feet on the dashboard and perform no discernable function whatsoever."

"I'm used to the journey; quite familiar with at least half of it. We'll get ourselves a coffee in Much Wenlock and have a little wander there before we start the foray into Wales. Always helps to break it ...."

Alex missed the end of the sentence as Jenny stepped through into the Ladies toilet. She was anxious about how Jenny might be feeling just now, suspecting a lingering psychological wound at the memory of abusive sex, but knowing it was better not to investigate further. She stood outside somewhat awkwardly and wondered how she came to be here, in the middle of God Knows Where, while she waited for Jenny to emerge. She comforted herself with the thought that she would be back home with Dan by tomorrow evening, and then life would settle back into its normal, safe routine. This was a crusade, an adventure, a step towards recovery. It had to be done.

CHAPTER 5

Approaching Much Wenlock

"Well, where were we?" asked Alex once the car had again reached its cruising speed, accelerating past any of the A road's light traffic which was slow moving. The sky had brightened a little and the threat of rain seemed to have diminished but Alex's body had, by now, adapted to the inside of the car rather than to the outside, and its limitations had blunted her response to the passing countryside. She added with a giggle, "I don't mean geographically! I know we're heading for Bridgenorth, wherever that may be. I mean, where were we philosophically? We said we'd carry on with it once we were en route again."

"No idea!" replied Jenny blithely, glancing across at Alex before positioning her gaze back onto the road ahead.

"You might prefer me to shut up for a while?"

"No, no! I'm relying on you to keep me awake. Carry on! Don't mind my absence of intelligent response. I haven't got the psychobabble gift at the best of times, but definitely not when I'm driving. We've got about fifty five miles now to go before we get to Much Wenlock, and then we'll take an hour's break. We should get to Annie's before seven, all being well. Wouldn't be fun to arrive much later! I don't fancy our chances of finding the place in the dark."

"D'you think we'll get a bite to eat at that hour? If I remember Wales accurately, the hungry visitor was out of luck if in search of pub food at twilight." Alex grimaced slightly, recalling a forlorn experience, long ago, of evening hunger in a rain soaked Welsh town.

"Annie will set us right, I'm sure," replied Jenny. "She's bound to know of a local hostelry where sustenance of a sort will still be on the menu. The peas will probably be tinned, though."

"Tinned peas?" repeated Alex, in surprise. "Oh well – I don't mind them, actually. Way back in my student days, I lived on a daily lunch of one boiled egg and half a tin of peas, for weeks on end. I never minded the monotony of it, and it meant I had about £4 left each week, saving up for rail fares and the occasions when Liam and I needed a Bed and Breakfast at Camberley. He was paid a pittance of an allowance at Sandhurst and every penny of it went on ciggies and suitable clothing like cavalry twills and checked shirts. He had to get the right gear as soon as possible. It's strange to think that the choice of casual wear for officer-cadets was almost more restricted than their military uniforms."

"What about dress for camp followers? I can't imagine you kitted up in horsy outfits, Alex!"

"Well, there's a fairly dismal photo of me and Liam taken in Sandhurst grounds after a parade. His dad probably took it. Maybe it was at Liam's passing out parade, because his parents came over from Ireland for that. Anyway, there I am, togged out in a shocking pink, knee length coat, a scrunched satin, close fitting pink hat and lumpy white gloves – and this at the height of the miniskirt era! I don't really remember what county set girlfriends wore to look 'O.Q.' (officer quality, me dear!) but I expect that it involved expensive items of clothing, made from silk, cashmere, linen; that sort of thing. I think that was back in the days before charity shops really caught on, and therefore I hadn't got a hope of buying expensive clothes and carrying off that sort of style. I expect I just looked like a slightly scrubbed up peasant, which was, after all, what I was."

"So were there charity shops in the Sixties?" enquired Jenny. "I can't remember; I don't think I got clothes from there, but I wasn't flush with cash in those days either. It's hard to imagine I bought everything new. Perhaps we just had fewer clothes back then. Whatever I had, it was usually pretty skimpy. I suppose I wore ridiculously short skirts, though I didn't much like wearing 'em. You needed to be tall and leggy to carry them off, and I didn't qualify. Oh dear! Youth is so wasted on the young isn't it? All that insecurity about our noses or ankles or bums and yet compared to how we are now......!" Jenny nodded down sadly towards her waist area, and Alex patted her own stomach in sympathy, sighing in agreement.

"Yes, I fussed endlessly about the odd spot on my face, my lack of cleavage and my lumpy knees, but most of all, about my frizzy hair. It was all a sort of vanity, really. How conceited of me to think that anyone else was bothered enough to register it. I suppose people notice my hair now all right! A long clump of tangled white frizz on the head of a middle aged woman seems to gain an occasional startled second look, despite my earnest hair band engineering. I used to be so jealous of all those girls with straight teeth and shiny hair which stopped suddenly. Ah! Jealousy! Now wasn't that what we were on about earlier? Narcissists and jealousy?"

Jenny glanced at her watch briefly. "You said something about envy being a key feature of Narcissists but I have to say, I don't remember either Joe or Ricky ever being jealous about me with other men. Not that I was going with any other men, of course, but if a man paid me a bit of attention, it was never an issue to either of them. So I don't really get this jealousy bit as a fundamental Narcissist emotion. I myself had a huge problem with it, of course, when Joe left with his leggy young model.

"But it felt much worse, all these years later, when Ricky sailed away to his Spanish mistress. I was so very, very angry and hurt and humiliated that he must obviously have thought so little of me. I found out much later that he had actually been discussing his dilemma of the choice between me and the new mistress for a year and a half, mulling it over with an old girlfriend of his in Ireland, keeping secrets and hiding things from me, who was supposed to be his partner and his best friend. I know we were having a rough time during that period – his job changes, my own stress levels, the lack of a stable base – but we might have been able to surmount our problems, even his infidelity, if we had only discussed them together. As it was, when I found out, he couldn't handle any sort of honest communication about it at all.

"It was incomprehensible, and it still is. Why did he just chuck the whole relationship away? Why do they do that? I was simply devastated to realise I could have been so wrong about someone I believed in. I was beside myself because of what might have been, and the careless way he blew it all. For a while, I was just transfixed with rage – I wanted to saw off his willie! Does that make *me* a Narcissist, then?"

Alex had to straighten her face before replying, "Well, we are all self absorbed and self protective to some extent, and there can be very few of us who could be at ease about suddenly losing a partner to someone else. It might be called 'Situational Narcissism', I suppose, bitterly to resent the loss of someone precious to you that you thought was in some way 'yours'. Anger and bitterness and jealousy seem appropriate enough as initial responses in that situation, but I think most of us can work down to a primary emotion of sadness in time. I think if we were never self centred in the sense of making our own needs high priority inwardly, we might be out of touch with the rest of humanity because we weren't even tuned in to ourselves.

"If we had set out on this trip, for example, Jenny, enthused with altruistic fervour to rescue Annie, but without eating or drinking or taking any breaks on our journey, we might arrive at her place quite incapable of helping anyone, since we hadn't looked after our own needs. Indeed, poor old Annie would be under pressure to rescue us instead, by providing for us what we didn't supply to ourselves."

"Well, I still don't get why my Narcissists weren't prone to jealousy when you say Narcissists are riddled with it. Was Liam the jealous type? Or Marcus?"

"Well, Liam certainly used to be paranoid that I might be eyeing up a man in mixed company, or vice versa. He was absolutely beside himself if ever his dad and mum were staying with us. There was some underlying hatred and rivalry between Liam and Gerry which I could never fathom. Maybe it was territorial – a father and first born son thing. Liam was utterly convinced his dad was trying to get off with me. I don't know where on earth it came from. It could have been because his dad was so jealous of Liam. After all, the golden boy was adored by his mum and older sister, got a decent education and eventually, even officer status which were all the things that his dad himself was denied. Maybe Liam just assumed that Gerry would naturally try to spite him in revenge, by pulling me.

"Anyway, whenever his mum and dad were over from Ireland on a visit with us, I would be firmly instructed to avoid finding myself alone with Gerry at any point, either inside or outside the house. Gerry, of course, had absolutely no desire to be in my company anyway, so that wasn't really a problem to me. Yet oddly enough, I don't think that Liam was jealous in the more normal sense of the word. He just wanted to make sure he had complete control over my actions so that any other bloke on the scene would recognise I wasn't 'up for it' elsewhere, which would, I suppose, be a terrible shame up for Liam. Oh, that's another essential element, as well as envy, they say: a total inability to handle any sort of shame.

"Marcus – no, I don't think he was ever jealous in the sense of seeing another man as a rival. He was actually pretty certain that every single woman he met was totally smitten by him! I remember when he first met Dan – oh, I think I've told you this before; sorry!"

Jenny shook her head briefly which signalled to Alex that she could carry on.

"He later informed me that he picked up a haunted expression in Dan's eyes as he shook hands with Marcus, an expression which Marcus interpreted as 'This is the man who is going to take away my wife from me.' Much later, I asked Dan about his first impressions of Marcus on that occasion, and he told me it was something along the lines of 'Bogus little shit!' coupled with instantaneous aversion."

"Oh, I do like Dan!" laughed Jenny. "No getting jealous or shamed up as far as he's concerned – just instant recognition of Marcus for what he was. If only our antennae could have been so finely tuned, we would have saved ourselves a lot of heartache. So why do we fall for these wazzocks when someone like Dan can recognise them instantly?"

"Well, I think it's because a Narcissist can intuitively sense whether the person in front of them is susceptible to his charms or not. Assuming that Marcus could see that Dan was neither impressed by his brain power nor attracted to his appearance, he wouldn't bother to turn on anything more than superficial politeness. However, he might well project his own latent jealousy and suspicion on to the other, since he does not allow himself to feel those sort of negative emotions personally. Thus, in Marcus's mind, he sees himself as being magnanimously courteous in the face of Dan's thinly veiled hostility. But when a predator like Marcus meets a susceptible person, he behaves very differently."

"Well, I didn't consider myself at all susceptible at first, either with Joe or with Ricky," remarked Jenny. "I told you how reluctant I was to interact with Joe when we met in Africa, and, in fact, my reaction to him wasn't unlike Dan's to Marcus, without the 'little'.

"And I was deeply distrustful of Ricky right from the start, and showed it. He first chatted me up on an Arts Council outing and I liked him well enough, but never thought he'd take it further than that day at the Ellison Statue Park. Then, much to my surprise, he sent me a birthday card addressed to the school because we hadn't exchanged home addresses or anything; something we'd talked about must have accidentally provided him with the upcoming date. (Hey, that's a Marcus technique isn't it? The surprise logging of a birth date!) Anyway, several weeks later, I sent a bland postcard to his work when I was on holiday. It wasn't until that autumn that we were accidentally in touch again. That was when he suggested arranging a meeting, and it quickly picked up from there.

"Within a couple of months, he had moved in with me, paying his share financially and enriching the quality of my life immeasurably. It didn't take long for me to feel that he had brought me alive in the most spectacular way. He had that amazing zest for life, for art, for all that was going on around us, especially culturally. He seemed so totally different from Joe who was, by then, said to be reduced to living in a rented bed sit on his own, balding, double chinned and a few stones heavier, aimlessly on the prowl for the next woman who might supply his various increasingly bizarre needs.

"I don't think I had felt in the least aimless or dreary when Ricky first came into my life. I'd been getting on quite happily with my work and my friends and with Julie and Matt launching themselves into careers, riding the inevitable thrills and spills alongside them. I wasn't 'looking for love' when I met Ricky, or back when I met Joe, for that matter. Both men in their turn bothered to make all the running at first, not me. So doesn't that upset your susceptibility theory?"

"Hmmm, yes, perhaps 'susceptible' is the wrong word. I think it actually goes back to this envy/shame thing in Narcissists, although

I admit I'm pretty confused by it all. Maybe what Narcissists sense is the opportunity for a kind of additional self protection? Women generally don't shame up men who are charming and attentive to them, even if certain women don't lap up the actual attention itself, but there's always the odd woman who might do the humiliation thing on him. So a Narcissist chooses just when to put his headlights onto full beam because he will not take kindly to a sharp reminder to dip his lights. He will see that oncoming light flashing as an agonising humiliation.

"Severe embarrassment isn't pleasant for anyone, but to a Narcissist it's annihilating. They feel exterminated by the slightest whiff of shame, and yet at some level, they are aware that they mysteriously seem to run the risk of behaving in a way that others consider to be 'shameful'. Their dysfunction means that they are bound to be seen as plonkers at times, and it must be pretty horrible for them to know this without having the skills to avoid it, or to handle it with self deprecating amusement if they do drop a real clanger. I think they are drawn to any person who could be flattered into providing psychological protection against their disgracing themselves in some way in the eyes of others."

"But I never gave either of my Narcissists the idea that I could protect them from embarrassment," protested Jenny. "*I* was the one far more likely to cause embarrassment because I tended to do things impulsively and say things off the top of my head. I'm afraid I seem quite at home with shame, one way or another."

"But that's it, Jenny! A Narcissist wants you as a protective shield. *You* aren't running scared from shame. You accept that it's inevitable, from time to time, that we might appear to let ourselves down in front of others, and we need to be resilient and recover from it. If we can handle shame that well, we probably were introduced to it in gentle doses, monitored by benign parents, at a very young age. It isn't such an issue for us, though of course nobody likes being shamed up.

"If we're lucky, I think we have a sort of immunity from the worst of it, because of those early controlled injections of it. If you wet the bed as a five year old, back then, you probably felt bad about it and didn't like the cold, damp smelliness of it, and might even be sorry for Mum having to wash the sheet. But you weren't made to feel disgusting or unlovable because of it. Nor would it have been hushed up, as if it was totally unmentionable in its horror. It was handled sort of in proportion – usually, anyway. Whereas I think for a Narcissist, those little shame ups of childhood were either hugely exaggerated, or assiduously covered up or even, in some cases, totally disregarded because the child was cosseted to believe he could do just as he liked at all times.

"Sometimes, if one parent loathes the child and the other adores him, the kid actually gets two of these disproportionate responses perpetually working in contrast to each other. I think Liam's dad always sought to exaggerate any social boob his young son made, whereas his mum and older sister constantly stroked and affirmed him in every way they could – perhaps in compensation? It seems a lethal combination to me, because later, the kid will be bemused as to which is the more skilful response to one's own social bog ups: to see a mistake as totally unforgivable, or to discount it entirely, projecting any circumstantial blame onto someone else. A happy medium between these two – acknowledgement coupled with learning about other possible choices for next time – is virtually impossible. But I do think Narcissists can recognise that 'happy medium' ability in others and seek to harness it for themselves."

"Well, I've never thought much about shame but I suppose it could have more significance than I give it. It's not a concept I've heard talked about much." Jenny reached for her water bottle and Alex unscrewed the lid for her, handed it over, and reversed the process once Jenny had gulped down several mouthfuls. Jenny nodded her thanks before speaking again, eyes on a van cutting in close ahead of her.

"I was always intrigued that neither Joe nor Ricky ever seemed to feel any guilt about anything, whereas I'm riddled with it! But I think guilt is about being personally responsible for things going wrong, whereas shame is maybe more to do with public perception. What about jealousy, then? You said that is supposed to be rampant in Narcissists, but as I said, it wasn't my experience."

"Ah, but I think each of your two men probably envied you, Jenny, without either you or he being aware of it. Perhaps there's the same sort of distinction between jealousy and envy as you just made between guilt and shame. Jealousy, like guilt, seems to me to be about a personal response to a specific trigger. But I think there may be an unconscious deep resentment of others' good fortune in the idea of envy; it's about feeling profoundly disadvantaged. I'm not sure but to me, the notion of jealousy seems to come from personal vulnerability in a particular situation. Does that make sense?"

"Are you suggesting that Narcissists operate from an envious position almost by definition?"

"Yes, I think I am. Envying others is, I think, the same thing as fearing them and feeling angry at what you perceive to be their potential advantage over you. Pathological envy means you feel entitled to destroy those others to establish your advantage over them instead. Hitler was good at fanning up murderous envy of the Jews but I don't think any Nazi would accept being described as jealous of the Jews. It's an odd coincidence, by the way, isn't it, that the words Narcissist and Nazi sound so alike!"

Jenny considered this for a moment before commenting, "No connection though – totally different roots; a Greek myth in one case, with its hero, Narcissus, as the beautiful, self absorbed young man, and a handily abbreviated German nickname for a National Socialist, in the other. But actually, from what you were saying, both Narcissists and Nazis have shame and envy as a central operational mode, haven't they? I mean, the likes of Hitler felt shamed up by the Allies at the end of the First World War, and there was also latent envy of the financial and social solidarity in Jewish society. Come to think of it, shame and envy probably lie at the heart of any oppressive movements. Could the grand "isms" – racism, imperialism, sexism – just be broader versions of Narcissistic Personality Disorder?

"That's quite a theory! I've never thought about that, but it makes sense. I certainly think Nazi theory and practice could be called 'Institutionalised Narcissism'," replied Alex, positioning one foot up on the dashboard. "It doesn't appear to be difficult to get a whole nation to act from a narcissist position, especially if you are as charismatic a leader as dear old Hitler. Hard to believe he was that much of a crowd drawer, though. He looks demented to me, when you see him on film."

"Those rallies were impressive, though; fantastic crowd management!" commented Jenny. "All that symbolic artwork was emotive stuff. There was a lot of spin doctoring going on, and it was incredibly effective. As far as I know, the swastika was a symbol which Hitler appropriated from Ancient Greece. So perhaps there *is* a Greek/Nazi link after all! It's very clever, isn't it, to promote a mystical, historic cultural identity through emotive symbols reproduced all over the place? That sort of hyped up climate is exactly what you need to twist the population's passionate responses into a fury of racial cleansing."

"And individual Narcissists do just the same thing," added Alex, warming to this theme. "Impressive flag waving, charismatic delivery, a destabilised surrounding ethos, the subtle use of shame and envy to discount the human rights of targeted others, and eventually taking a course of action which leads to devastation all round. Stalin, Hitler, Mao, Amin – weren't they actually all Malignant Narcissists who left mass slaughter in their wake?

"But our own four civilised Narcissists are just as destructive in their own much more limited spheres; look what havoc they have achieved in our shattered minds! It's just that their currency is in psychological ambushes rather than in mass graves. I admit I was pretty barmy in the first place, but I wasn't mentally obliterated until 'Marcus aftershock' kicked in. I knew something odd was happening in my head but I wouldn't acknowledge it. So very, very stubborn and stupid of me – I thought I could handle it!" Alex sighed and shook her head slightly. There was a pause before a connected thought struck her.

"You know, I always felt sympathy for Neville Chamberlain returning from that meeting with Hitler in 1938 and waving the piece of paper which said, 'Peace in Our Time!' or something. I used to watch a lot of War documentaries as a teenager for some reason. It was probably because I couldn't think of anything else to do on dreary Sunday afternoons! Anyway, poor old Chamberlain was ridiculed later, after Hitler invaded Poland, but God! I understand so well that feeling of elation he must have had; that we're bringing out the best in people, not the worst. It seems strange that in dealing with one particular section of humanity, that sort of trusting optimism actually ceases to be a virtue and becomes sheer, blind pigheadedness. Chamberlain paid heavily for his gullibility, and Churchill, the ultimate War Lord, finally got his chance for leadership. You and I have managed to make the same mistake as Chamberlain twice and, in a way, we got war in our heads as a result."

Alex was unsure whether this sort of analysis was nonsensical. She glanced over towards Jenny, who was quiet for a few seconds before switching the topic of conversation slightly.

"But it's so much worse this time than it was for me after Joe – why is that? Is it because second time round, it has built up to hurt far more?"

"Hmm. It's the same with me," sighed Alex, still playing with her wedding ring absently. "Yep, I think it might be insidious accumulation of damage, Jenny, as you say; a bit like the third bee sting can cause someone anaphylactic shock because – er – is it that the immune system becomes disabled dealing with the first two, however long the intervals were in between?

"Or perhaps, as we said, the first time, we hadn't got a chance of dealing with the full impact of it, with two young kids to look after. Or were we just more resilient at 30 than we are in our 50's? We believed we were young enough to recover and make a new life for ourselves then, and for the new opportunities to restore us. This time, we've had to work at recovery from the inside out, rather than the outside in. Maybe that's why it's so much tougher. We are, at last, facing up to a crisis that we dodged all those years ago. Mind you, Jenny, you've said before that you seriously thought of topping yourself after Joe left. Surely things couldn't have felt much worse than that? It's hardly dodging the enormity of your pain to be working out how to give yourself a lethal dose of carbon dioxide in a car."

"Yes, I was pretty determined to do myself in at one point. That phase passed quite rapidly, though, when I realised it was impractical, given the complications of two young kids left alone in the house. The logistics of suicide perplexed me. If I left a note for a neighbour before I drove off to do the deed, it might be found too soon, and I'd be embarrassingly rescued, or too late, in terms of the kids having a considerable time on their own in the house to rush about in a panic. I couldn't really think of a solution. So I eventually gave up on the idea."

"Thank the Lord for pragmatism!" smiled Alex, hands outstretched. "Knowing you, you would have performed the whole operation with efficient success, if the complexities of immediate childcare hadn't stopped you. Oh Jenny! To take away your own life permanently when, in fact, Joe had only appeared to destroy it temporarily; that would have been tragic irony indeed! I'm so glad you came out of that for everyone's sake, and especially for mine, by the way, my dear mate in catastrophe and turmoil!"

There was a brief pause. Jenny found such spontaneous expressions of warmth disconcerting, although she was also touched by them. She glanced at her watch and remarked briskly, "We're doing well, time wise; only about ten miles to go before our next break. We'll be able to get coffee and a loo. It may not be a thriving industrial metropolis but Much Wenlock has all the necessities of life, garnished with Olde Worlde charm. It'll be good to have a brief dander, too, in the fresh air." She paused before adding, "What about you then, Alex? Were you ever suicidal?"

"I think I toyed with the idea of it; once or twice at boarding school in dear ol' Dublin, and then again, after Liam left. But I don't think it was more than a passing thought in my mind. Somehow, I developed a rather censorious attitude to suicide pretty early in my life – suicide caused by a wounding psychological experience, anyway. If someone was in tremendous physical pain, or had lost all hope of any quality of life, that's different, but I suppose I have something of the Scarlet O'Hara philosophy: 'Tomorrow is Another Day' and all that.

"It seemed to me that people sometimes commit suicide to show someone else what awful hurt he or she caused. That would appear to be impractical as a revenge gesture since, if you've gone and killed yourself, you wouldn't actually be around to savour the other person's agonised guilt!

"And that's another thing about suicide: it looks like a huge circle of your relations and friends and associates will be permanently traumatised by your doing yourself in, and that your nearest and dearest will simply never get closure on your death. It seems pretty crappy to cause such shockwaves of devastation when, if you'd just waited a bit, things might have improved, in a week or a month or a year.

"And.... there's yet another argument against it – a bit cooky this one! In my erstwhile metaphysical exploratory phase, I read somewhere that an embodied soul that has destroyed its physical form comes to awareness in the Great Beyond and – guess what! – feels exactly as it did just before it did the dastardly deed. Suicide wouldn't be much of a solution in that event. You still have to work through the crisis, but now you have to do it without physical embodiment, which is a further challenge, and has actually just made recovery even harder. Neat, isn't it? I like that argument!"

"You'd make a rotten Samaritan, Alex, with that wodge of anti suicide spin. Mind you, I had to resign from the 'Sams' myself! It wasn't that I wanted to present arguments against suicide, though. I just felt that a lot of the people who were ringing weren't in the sort of situation where talking or being listened to would make any difference either way."

"How d'you mean?"

"Well, I think maybe there are so many ways that relatively sane people can gain help to work through a crisis nowadays – agencies, self help books, doctors referrals, support groups, all that sort of thing – that quite a few of those who are reduced to repeatedly ringing a Samaritan Helpline when they feel low are almost beyond constructive help. I think some doctors actually tell such patients to give us a ring us because they know we're a last resort, as a sort of 'help for the helpless'. It seemed to me that the majority of my callers – well, the men, anyway – were stuck in a cycle of heavy breathing, wanking off, or just ritual reciting of dirty deeds done against them. Basically, they were people with on going mental health issues, and nothing I could provide for them would make any difference."

"That sounds familiar!" laughed Alex. "You and I seem to be fatally drawn towards trying to redeem men who have serious mental health issues. Your phone line wanker is surely just a much more basic version of our own dear Narcissists? (Different currency, again: not psychological ambushes this time, but sticky tissues!) And if that's the case, you were quite right to resign from an organisation which continues to collude with them!"

"Well, in fairness, 'Sams' doesn't encourage stuck interactions with clients. There were immediate sign off routines if we suspected our voices were being used for masturbation purposes. For those clients who talked unceasingly, reworking the same litany of ills, time and time again, there were other procedures. We would have case meetings about that sort of client, who invariably make the same sort of call repeatedly, whoever the responding 'Sam' may be. Usually, the conclusion was that the contact with them should be limited, and that they should be informed of the restrictions with gentle courtesy. 'Now, Larry, we are reaching your limit of phone time for the week – two twenty minute calls – so we will need to finish within five minutes. Is there any last thing you'd like to share before we sign off for now?' That sort of thing. Curiously, there is rarely any objection from the caller. Often, he seems almost touched by the apparent significance of his calls and the thought that there is an established set of rules about communication with him as an individual. It gives him a sort of identity, perhaps...... I dunno."

"Is it difficult to specify that sort of discipline thing, though? To break into their ramblings with a line as directive as that?"

"No, not really. It's a bit like telling the kids at school that it's time to pack away the equipment, five minutes before the bell. But I began to find that the stuckness of some 'Sams' clients' mental state still lingered with me, and it might weigh down my mind days later when I was wheeling a shopping trolley or changing a light bulb or something. And I didn't like that impact one bit. So I thought I'd better write in to the headquarters and say I needed a break from 'Sams' for a while and that I would contact them once I was up for it again. They were very understanding. But I don't think I'll return to it. Somehow, it just isn't right for someone like me." Jenny shrugged slightly, as if resigned to this conclusion.

"Oh, I don't think it's about 'someone like you' – it's not a personality thing!" Alex protested. "It's surely about where we are at? And at the moment, maybe our first priority is to work our way out of our own stuckness over Ricky and Marcus. Perhaps that's why the stuckness of some of those clients haunted you; you recognised that you yourself felt somehow boxed into some dark corner, like me, even if, superficially at least, you were coping pretty efficiently with your life."

"But how *do* we work our way out of it, Alex? I still don't know how to do it – not a clue. Every time I think I'm coming out of the tunnel, I seem to plunge back into darkness again. I often think I am never ever going to get back to how I was before. I can't get over the unanswerable lament of 'Why?' That question haunts me a lot of my time. Why did it all go so wrong and get rubbished so carelessly when the relationship was to me one of genuine connection? That's true for both Joe and Ricky, from my point of view. Is it something wrong with me, that I eventually push them away subconsciously, or that I'm just not good to be with, after they really get to know me? It all goes round and round in my mind and batters me, even in my sleep. I simply can't understand why it happened. I just don't get it!"

Alex glanced across at Jenny in some concern. Not for the first time, she wondered if it was actually harming Jenny further to foist endless analytical explorations onto her so often when they met.

"Well…" she hesitated, biting her lower lip. "Well, – maybe, dear Jenny, we will never get back to how we were before. But perhaps that's good? Because before, we were very vulnerable to 'Being of Service to Narcissists'. We saw our pragmatic, resourceful mums doing it all through our childhoods, and doing it very skilfully for our Public Figure dads. It seemed to work out pretty well. My mum did it, but still had her archaeology and her social networks; your mum did it but still had her good works, and her arty craftiness and her three girls – bringing you up was her domain, wasn't it? And she cornered your dad right out of it. But you and I don't seem to have the special sort of talent that our mums had; to play the admiring, devoted supporter, while retaining our own identity."

Jenny thought about this for a moment before picking up the theme. "Maybe there's the additional factor that our mums were toughened by their own early upbringing: mine in the Canadian Outback, yours in India, wasn't it, before landing up in Northern Ireland? You and I had less cultural upheaval as kids than our mothers did, and had a more stable base, I suppose. So maybe we weren't adequately toughened? Somehow, we eventually let ourselves be swallowed up by our Narcissists instead.

"But then, our mums may have basically been just stronger types than us? More self reliant and less in search of soul intimacy? Was that a cultural thing, d'you think? They were products of their time, the war and all that, whereas we are the Baby Boomer generation who had it easy and wants it all; Flower Power Peace and Love, Commitment and Everlasting Soul Mate Connection in Loving Relationships, Financial Comfort, A Good Pension, A Saved Planet, Long term Good Health, and A Cosy, Painless Death, well beyond our three score years and ten?"

"Hmmm, yes, I think you're certainly right that our mothers didn't expect their partner also to be their soul mate and their best friend," Alex responded. "But maybe our own Narcissists were simply much more damaging in relationship than either of our fathers? Maybe it was a combination of the two? It's a mystery." She shook her head briefly, with a slight shrug.

"I certainly think my mum was a lot tougher than me, in that she always knew what her own standpoint was," remarked Jenny, engrossed in this line of investigation. "She knew she was the power behind the throne, as far as Dad was concerned. She was much more resilient than he was. Survival in the coldness of the Canadian Outback must have been quite a struggle for her own family when they first went out there, without either money or due preparation for the severe challenge of the environment. So she knew all about the fight for survival from the age of three. She wasn't warm, pink and fluffy, and she didn't encourage us to be, either.

"She certainly wasn't a sentimental mum, but if the chips were down, she was there with all the practical support she could provide, before you even asked for it. Not long after Joe left, she came to stay with me for a fortnight because Julie had had a burst appendix and was really very ill. Mum's rapid response tactics leapt into action when she assessed the local hospital's standards of care, and within two days she was nursing Julie back to health at home with me."

"So which type of mum are we, then?" asked Alex. "Are we the tough, resourceful mums, always ready with practical help, or the warm pink fluffy ones, always boosting the little darlings' morale through devoted empathy? And which should we be?"

"Sometimes we need to be one, and sometimes the other, and sometimes a subtle combination of the two. And at other times we have to step back completely. It's a question of being attuned to the signals, I suppose, so that there can be a constant feedback loop between mum and kid. Maybe that's another symptom of rapidly falling prey to Narcissists, Alex? If we are used to tuning in with adaptive empathy to our own kids' needs, especially our sons', does that mean that male Narcissists, who are really just manipulative little chaps emotionally, Peter Pans, can tug at our heart strings at the very deepest level of our nurturing instincts?"

"......So that when the Narcissist then abandons us, it is somehow as devastating as the death of a little son? Come to think of it, losing a child seems to be among the most profound of all possible losses; it looks as if it's one that people never really get over. Wow! Jenny, I think you're on to something there!" Alex hugged her knees in excitement, grinning wildly. *"That's* why we coped better with being annihilated first time round – because each of us had at least one little male offspring still on our hands to nurture, even after our dear husband's departure. You're a janius!"

"Wait a minute! How? What did I say?" Jenny glanced across at Alex with a bemused twitch of the mouth, her arms momentarily stretched straight out on either side of the steering wheel.

"Well, let's suppose that we are programmed to nurture our young, for the preservation of our genes, and all that. Surely that must be the case? Then to nurture and subsequently to be cut off from the very being we nurtured must be a severe trauma for us. I suppose it's like realising we were lavishing our worms on a cuckoo chick!"

"But the cuckoo chick doesn't intend any harm to its adoptive nurturers, does it?" Jenny tried to remember what she knew about this aspect of bird behaviour, with some difficulty. "Its parents just borrowed other birds' nests for their own young. I suppose the egg shell's colour and patterning must be similar to the host birds' eggs, to fool the nest owners. Anyway, the cuckoo parents have simply delegated the feeding process. I expect they only have a short breeding time available, but maybe the female can produce quite a few eggs during the spring and early summer, before they're off to warmer climes again. Seems quite crafty if the parents can get more eggs reared by using a series of unwitting fosterers to incubate one egg at a time for them. It's not the egg's fault if it's dumped on fosterers, is it?"

"Ah, but the little cuckiboos will get too big to share food or the nest space! And I think that when they hatch, they use their backs somehow to shunt the host parents' own fledglings out of the nest. I think it's something like that. The cuckoo chick gradually gets to take over the whole space within the nest. Given that it's much bigger than the host birds' chicks, this has to happen if the cuckoo is to survive. You're right that it's the nest borrowing by the cuckoo parents which results in their chick thriving at the expense of the smaller resident fledglings. It wouldn't make sense, though, to say that the cuckoo fledgling plots to eject his adoptive siblings; it's surely an essential adjunct to his parents' nurturing style. Hey, how about that for a dissertation title: 'The Cuckoo Parent as Narcissist; a detailed study of the pathological exploitation of the ornithological nurturing instinct '? I like it!"

Both women chuckled briefly. Then Jenny frowned slightly in concentration, evidently puzzled.

"But surely it can't be pathological if it's a natural instinct within the world of birdery? Isn't it just something cuckoos do? It's the same sort of thing as those large visually impaired female spiders who are quite likely to gobble up their little mates after sex, mistaking them for intruders on their space. If it isn't intended to be malicious, it must just be an adaptive mode of survival which works effectively for that particular creature, however weird it seems to us humans."

"Well, now we're entering the subtleties of what's natural and what's pathological. Is it in some animals' nature to usurp the territory of others or to exploit their nurturing, or even to eat their own lovers or family members? I suppose we have to say that it is.

"And human beings are just sophisticated animals. So, presumably, we as a species may also reflect that basic programming to usurp, exploit and destroy. But as human beings have evolved, over vast stretches of time, we have eventually come to investigate how to move above and beyond that, haven't we? If we didn't have reasoning to allow us to select some survival strategies rather than those ones, our species would surely have been wiped out ages ago. Some forms of group cooperation must have gradually emerged as the technique which works best for primates. It appears to be a key survival strategy in ever changing environments.

"Come to think of it, there must be many creatures who work on a cooperative principle for the efficiency of the community – like bees or ants, for example. So there are all sorts of survival strategies available. It's just that humans seem to have developed the capacity to pick and mix among those choices, according to the resources and threats in their environment."

"But can we really pick and mix?" Jenny was still frowning slightly. "I mean, human beings have markedly different personalities and resources and cultural environments, and there are many contrasting ways in which various societies interpret the drives which govern human behaviour, whether the terminology is about magical protection against demonic possession or about flexible versus rigid defence systems. Surely some human beings have very little choice at all? You can see their vulnerability most clearly in war zones or in the plight of victims who have been denied the fair distribution of survival resources like water, food and shelter, worldwide. Their plight doesn't result from any choice of theirs."

"But the truth is that even privileged people in the most favourable environments may have dire restrictions on their power to choose," Alex replied swiftly. "Rich parents don't necessarily empower their children to make the choices which will best suit their healthy psychological development. And there are biological defence systems lodged within our bodies that can run amok and cause our immune system to attack itself. In the same way, psychological defence systems can take over our minds to create a horrific nightmare scenario out of the most mundane of incidents.

"I read somewhere that it isn't the cold virus itself which is so unpleasant; it is the body going into overdrive to defend itself against the virus – blocked nose, aching sinuses and all that – which produces symptoms much worse than what is actually being defended against. In the same way, the interpretation of danger conceived by a mind in the grip of some extreme sort of paranoia is almost certainly more lethal than any genuine threat which may exist in the environment.

To arm yourself against an attack by a random stranger and to defend yourself by stabbing him to death when he had only been trying to hurry past you on the pavement to catch his bus; that's a good example, isn't it? In that sort of case, the nature of the paranoid defence action is far more violently destructive than the real encounter.

"So another factor in whether we can pick and mix between defence strategies is our level of awareness; our ability to see things as they really are. Consciousness is the same as awareness, I suppose. I think that's what allows each of us, again and again, to make a choice on defence matters, according to the immediate situation which confronts us.

"In my years of trying to make sense of things after Liam left, I eventually got hold of Krishnamurti's books. He was an Indian teacher, famous in the Thirties, an international speaker but determinedly non guru. He used to lecture in one of his educational headquarters during one week every summer, and I used to go down from London to Hampshire to hear him speak. I think I did that three years running, if I remember rightly. It was all very ecologically sound, like a wholesome Buddhist picnic, with absolutely no hype whatsoever. At a given time, this slight figure would slip in through a flap in the marquee and seat himself on a wooden chair. He was, by this time, a frail old man with a lot of white hair and a face etched with a harsh sort of compassion. He'd talk quietly to the assembled audience for an hour and then glide out again, to no applause. You'd be hard put to it, later, to summarise what he had said or taught; perhaps that's because he was somehow just presenting us with a way to *be*.

"He was against all organised belief systems, and up for Truth being a Pathless Land. His philosophy was all about the Freedom we might find when we ditch fear and just go for awareness. One of the titles of his books was, 'Freedom, Love and Action'. The word order is interesting, there. He was on about how each of us has to undergo a sort of psychic revolution within our own consciousness, in order to have genuine freedom of choice. No other species demonstrates that ability, in theory, because only human beings have the material of consciousness to work on."

"Well, can *we* do that?" asked Jenny, with interest. "You and me, I mean. Is our level of awareness well enough attuned to see things with our Narcissists as they really are?"

"No, I don't think it is, but we're working on it," replied Alex, with a brief smile. "Once, in our youth, our awareness level was far too low and we were swept along, delighted to be providing the vehicle for someone else's dreams. Now, I think we've probably tipped much too far the other way! We seem to be obsessively hyper vigilant about the whole matter of intimate relationship; maybe a sort of havoc romping through our psychological immune system. You could call it 'Reactive Lupus' in our wiring! It feels like insanity – white noise in the soul. But I'd like to believe it's a natural stage which we can move through eventually, if we allow ourselves to experience it fully. We can't bypass it or reason ourselves out of it because the wiring which might conceivably allow us to carry out such a strategy is impaired by the condition itself.

"The worst thing to do is to condemn ourselves for being in the state at all, or to become more afraid of the state than of the original damage done to us by our contact with a pretender. We should thank our inbuilt defence systems most courteously for seeking to look after us in this radically proactive way, and applaud their dedication. Once we cease to be full of fear and self loathing about it, there is far more chance that our wiring can begin to restore itself and function more healthily. Then, as old K.M. would have it, we'd experience Freedom, and we'd be able to Love (healthily, of course, through awareness!) and put that Love into Action. The most useful thing of all is to choose to surround ourselves with other people who are also searching for a mentally healthy route to survival."

"But mentally healthy people can be so dull!" wailed Jenny, with a chuckle of despair. "How can we cope with the sepia of Order in relationship when we've been on the thrilling Disorder roller coaster for so long? Being sensibly grounded is unbearably pedestrian! It feels like sinking into monochrome after soaring in glorious technicolour. I think I may have got addicted to danger over the years, and part of me still craves another fix of it."

Jenny twitched her shoulders slightly in resignation. The traffic ahead of her was beginning to slow down as they approached the town limits. She sniffed and remarked dolefully, "Ah well, I'll just have to sublimate my destructive urges by drinking strong coffee. This is Much Wenlock, by the way, tra la la! We'll park in the main drag and search out a café; okay?"

"Wonderful!" replied Alex, suddenly keen to be out of the car and on her feet. There were plenty of parking spaces in the main square since it was already after four o'clock, and the Saturday shoppers were thinning out in number. Both women were soon standing outside the locked car, breathing in a sharper, fresher sort of air.

"This way!" said Jenny with authority, and Alex hurried up alongside her to cross over the road and through the arch beneath the clock tower.

CHAPTER 6

Commercial Break

It seemed surprising that the shops were still available for browsing, even if only for a further hour, before the weekend shut down. A long car journey can put some passengers into a sort of no man's land where the choice of retail therapy, however brief, would seem like a glimpse of paradise to them. The sort of shopping now on offer was precisely the kind which appealed to both women, and within a few minutes they were exploring the covered market with its colourful variety of stalls and goods, remarking on the range of high quality and low priced fruit and vegetables for sale. Some of the stalls were closing down, but the area had not yet acquired the forlorn quality of dereliction which Alex always dreaded. Jenny bought some luscious looking cherries, handed over by a woman who used a sturdy brown bag as a container, and who delivered several expressions of endearment to her customer, in the process of filling it to the brim.

The accent of the man in the Antique/Junk shop over the road and up on the other side was somewhat similar to the fruit seller's, but his voice was much quieter, and he showed little interest in either his wares or his customers, preferring to linger in the dimness at the back of his narrow shop. Again, this suited the two women well, allowing them to browse through numerous random groups of objects, ranging from a moth eaten stuffed rodent of some kind to a small cream maker with a blue plastic pump handle.

"I'm always on the lookout for a paper knife," Jenny commented to Alex as she rummaged through a cracked jug crammed full of tarnished cutlery.

"A paper knife?" echoed Alex mindlessly. She had never used or owned one.

"Yes. I used to have a lovely little mother of pearl one, long ago, but it disappeared. I've never been able to replace it."

Alex glanced up at the shelves behind the glass counter ahead of them. There seemed to be more collections of cutlery upon them, as well as several other trays of miscellaneous objects, though it was hard to make this out in the dim light. She considered turning to ask the lurking figure beyond them whether they might look through the less accessible bundles of cutlery, but it proved to be unnecessary. He appeared to have caught the essence of their conversation, if not the actual wording.

"You lookin' for anything in particular?" he asked Jenny. There was a slight air of impatience about him, as if these tail end customers were an intrusion on his privacy.

"Yes; a paperknife," replied Jenny promptly.

He turned away from them and positioned himself behind the counter, disappearing from view as he dabbled among stacks of items, apparently at knee or ground level. Eventually, he reappeared with three small knives in his hand. He laid them on the counter without enthusiasm. They qualified as knives, certainly, but their handles were not decorated and there was little about them to suggest the elegant art of envelope opening. Alex peered down at them, registering that there was nothing fancy about their handles. Jenny, however, picked up the daintiest of the three and turned it over in her hand.

"Oh, I like this one!" she said. "How much is it?"

"Four pound. T'handle's bone."

"Yes, I'll have it, please."

Alex reached into her fleece pocket, misshapen by the weight of small change, and leant over to deposit four pound coins on the counter. Jenny looked over at her in surprise and then protested crossly, "Oh, Alex! Why should you pay for it? Honestly! You always do this, given half a chance."

"Jenny, it's nothing. Please let me! I haven't paid a penny towards petrol yet or anything."

"We agreed we'd sort out all that later. There's no need for you to finance any random whim of mine!"

The women hmffed at each other briefly. Meanwhile, the shopkeeper wrapped the little knife in a bit of crumpled tissue paper and then handed it over to Jenny, who was still clicking her tongue. Alex expected to be scolded further when they emerged into the street again, but Jenny seemed so pleased with the purchase that she switched to thanking Alex instead.

"Wonderfully symbolic, isn't it?" laughed Alex in relief, linking arms with Jenny for a moment. "We need a knife to cut the cords which bind us to our Narcissists, don't we? And I guess it also needs to be a joint ambition. It has never seemed possible to me to do it on my own."

"Me, neither!" nodded Jenny, with a sympathetic squeeze of arms. "Now, I noticed a café down that side street, Alex. Shall we see if they're still serving? I really could do with a bit more caffeine firing up my system before the last leg of the journey…."

"……when we hit darkest Wales?" Alex finished the sentence for her.

"Well, we're very close to Wales now, actually. But there's quite a long way to go once we cross the border, and it would be a relief to make it comfortably before seven. We're certainly more than half way. So we've 'broken the back of the journey', as my dear father would have put it. He had lots of little expressions like that, all to do with distances to be covered. He travelled a lot, of course, for his job. But, you know, however long the journey, he actually loved driving, and always played classical music in the car, wherever he went. I realise now how much he wanted one of us to enjoy his music alongside him. He was a truly cultured man, really, without being at all posh about it. Of course, we kids took no interest in his chosen music whatsoever. I know it would have touched him deeply if even one of us had; he was so rarely in a position to forge any connection with his three daughters who were so clearly the mother hen's chicks and not his territory."

"My dad was always keen to get 'the best of the day'; that was his key phrase. I expect our fathers would have liked one another, don't you think? And our mothers, too? They had lots in common, personality wise." Alex paused before continuing, "I remember Dad really loved people who Seized Their Opportunity, whatever that might be. One morning in the summer holidays, he went to this corrugated iron shed where one of the school workmen lived; an old Scotsman in a dark blue boiler suit who used to ring the school bell in the yard every morning in term time, among other jobs. Jock was his name; he was a dear man, but not that literate.

"Anyway, it was a gorgeous summer morning and Jock had pinned a note on his door which said, 'To fine – R out.' My dad really loved that! He so well understood the necessity to use that spectacularly beautiful day, not stay in on the off chance of a job needing to be done. 'Too fine – are out'! Dad told the story so many times! He was a great raconteur, of course, and Mum always laughed at his stories, however often she heard them. I think half the reason Dad's tales amused other people so much was that he was always choking with laughter as he told them, and that was kind of infectious. He was a natural performer, really. Your dad must have been even more so, to be so successful at the BBC. Maybe that's why we both became teachers, Jenny? Perhaps we weren't sufficiently extraverted to perform with enjoyment, but at least we had plenty of experience as children, watching how it was done."

"Yep – but in a way, sometimes that's a disadvantage, isn't it? We end up in a job we can do, and a job which is very amenable to our own kids' holidays, but we don't really stop to consider whether we are actually cut out for it! That's just the arrogance of being young and sure we can manage anything we set our minds to, I suppose. Oh, good! Here's the café, and it looks as if they're still serving all right."

They stepped into the entrance and took up a table near the centre of the room, as the window seats were already occupied. The café's layout and window frontage suggested that it had once been a shop, and this gave it a rather uncertain validity as an eating area. As if aware of this deficiency, the décor was determinedly cosy, in a busily floral decorative style. The predominant colours were black and pink, and each table had a small pink electric candle in its centre, dimly aglow. This illumination seemed surprising, given it was still broad daylight outside. Both women seated themselves and glanced round, trying to work out if they were supposed to go up to make an order or whether they would be served. The latter seemed more likely, given the aura of old fashioned quaintness about the place.

Sure enough, within a few minutes a young girl arrived to take their order, and it was not long before two large cappuccinos were carefully placed on the black table between them. They both smiled and nodded their thanks before the girl turned away. Their smiles were much broader, however, as she moved out of earshot.

"Well, just look at that!"

Jenny giggled as she indicated the frothy surface of her cup, and gestured towards the matching appearance of Alex's coffee.

"Perfect!" exclaimed Alex, with a grin of delight.

Jenny took the edge of her teaspoon and drew it diagonally across the chocolate sprinkled outline of a heart floating on top of the froth. Alex copied her immediately, pleased to see how her diagonal line of exposed coffee colour actually looked like part of the original symbol.

"Two bwoken hearted waifs, we are!" she laughed across the table. "Oh, Jenny, what are we like? Sad or what?"

"We're certainly sad, mad or bad – or maybe all three. But we are trying to be something different aren't we? 'Glad' would be the aim, I suppose. How's that for a strap line? "Not mad or bad or sad, but glad, glad, glad!"

"I like it!"

Both women whispered the phrase in rhythmic harmony, until Jenny caught a furtive glance in her direction from a nearby table. "That's enough for now, girls," she intoned primly, her tone school teacher clipped. "Settle down, please, and get on with your work."

Alex pulled her lips down, ducked her head, and they both slurped at their coffee in noisy unison.

Alex's feelings of insecurity were beginning to mount as the car sped towards the border between England and Wales. She had some memory of crossing this boundary before and a jumble of associations – scarily high bridge, money to pay, big river far down below them, suspension cables looming above – came to mind, but Jenny had abruptly banished them by declaring the border route they were taking to be totally unremarkable. Apparently, only one signpost on the left hand side signalled their arrival in Wales by bidding them a welcome in Welsh and then in English.

Alex looked out for any obvious signs of contrast in the landscape or traffic volume but again, there were none to speak of. However, she guessed that as they travelled deeper into the heart of the Welsh countryside, differences would become much more evident, particularly as, by then, evening would be approaching. Alex was unsettled by this thought, and glanced across at Jenny to reassure herself of the driver's unwavering confidence.

"How are we doing?" she asked, glancing down at the map on the floor near her feet.

"Oh, I'm fine for the next hour, I think," replied Jenny cheerfully. "I remember the route to Llangollen; it's perfectly straightforward: A5 all the way. Actually, we run parallel to Offa's Dyke from now on for most of the stretch to Annie's. It's a lovely area; very unspoilt, and hardly a soul in sight when you're walking. I had a lovely weekend here once. One night, I remember, I had an entire en suite dormitory all to myself in one of the Youth Hostels along the way.

"I came here the same year I met Ricky. We had encountered one another briefly that summer, and it was in response to that birthday card I told you about, the one he sent me at school, that I sent him the innocuous post card from my walk here. He then sent me an equally bland card from Ireland. It was not until October of that year when I rang the Arts Council office and found myself speaking to him, not the woman there I was supposed to contact, that we made an arrangement to meet up. It all seemed very random and unlikely." Jenny sighed and shook her head briefly, before carrying on.

"Anyway, Alex, once we turn off for Ruthin, I'll need you to attempt a bit of direction giving, but it will all be signed, anyway. And once we find ourselves in deepest, darkest Wales, we can refer to Annie's instructions. We're doing rather well, you know." Jenny tilted her head slightly, in appreciation of the distance covered.

"You must be getting tired, though, Jenny; it's a hell of a lot of driving."

"Well, I'll be glad to get there, but I don't feel tired at all at the moment. The coffee helps and so do your psychoanalytical wanderings, though I can't always make sense of them, of course. God knows how you waded through all those tomes of yours, Alex! I found those Self Help ones hard going enough, and I only read two of them. The pair of them must have been aimed at a mass market of those who know nuzzink about psychological dysfunction, yet the concepts can still be hard to get your head round. But you've trawled through countless volumes of the stuff at all levels! How on earth did you stick at it? And why?"

"I suppose it was a kind of obsession," sighed Alex, holding her forehead briefly in recollection. "After Marcus's sudden cut off, I so much needed to come to grips with what had happened to my head. I sort of kept hoping that one of the books would miraculously contain that one sentence which would suddenly make sense of it all. I'd already realised that I wasn't going to find a real living person who could straighten it out for me; neither conventional medicine nor psychic healing nor acupuncture, nor someone who trod all over me bones. (Shiatsu, is it?) You name it, I tried it, one after another, but although some of them helped a bit for a few hours, it never seemed to touch the long term damage.

"Eventually, I went back to my doctor for another course of antidepressants. He was puzzled about it; not surprisingly, poor man, as I told him nothing about Marcus. He had treated me for the depression which had carted me out of school three years previously, and he obviously couldn't quite work out why it had reappeared when I was now well clear of the teaching profession. He decided to refer me to a National Health psychiatrist, a chum of his, who was interested and sympathetic, and bent the rules a bit to give me two free sessions and one briefer follow up. (I was much more honest with her!) She couldn't give me more time than that because she said I wasn't bad enough; she had a huge waiting list, of course, and I was technically functional, after all. I also got myself a private counsellor, much later, who was really kind and supportive. I'm not knocking any of them. But I suppose I guessed that the answer – well, my answer – lay somewhere in one of these books, and I just had to read on until I found it. You had more sense than to waste your time on such stuff, Jenny."

"Not particularly more sense; I just had less of a drive to analyse myself and to search for answers. I dealt with the pain differently, I suppose; by blocking it out as far as possible. I expect that's why I felt like a hologram. If I wasn't feeling the pain, there wasn't much else of me left to feel anything. So I worked. I set myself projects, hurled myself at things – just kept as busy as possible which wasn't hard, really, since by then I was teaching full time at the Special Needs School. But free time was harder because all my creativity for my own art work was on hold. I didn't want to go back on antidepressants because they'd zombified me when I'd taken them long before all this, and now I seemed able to achieve the same spaced out effect on myself without medication.

"I don't think anybody noticed how I was, after a while. I think people close to me knew I was very angry about Ricky going off with Madeleine, but perhaps they thought I should have been prepared for it. He was, after all, a typical Irish charmer who had wheedled his way into sharing my home, given me eight years of his festive company without exploiting me financially, and then moved on to foreign fields with a new, younger love who could offer even more. We weren't actually married, and he hadn't conned me out of money or seduced my daughter......"

"But surely your own kids must have felt very hurt themselves? I mean, I know he wasn't exactly a father figure to them at their age, but they were fond of him, weren't they? He had been part of their lives, too, just as you had been for his kids, even if yours were in their late teens or 20's when you two first got together. Wasn't his youngest daughter only about thirteen when you met?"

"No, younger than that; Sandie was only just eleven. His three kids were based in Ireland with his ex, the singer, but they would come over and stay with him from time to time, or he would go back to Ireland and land himself on his clan, and bring his kids to join him there. Oh, look over there, Alex! Look at the colour of that distant horizon; it's sort of apricot, isn't it? Such vastness! I love the remoteness of it all!"

Alex nodded vaguely with a nervous glance over to the indicated distance, and waited for Jenny to carry on.

"Um – yes... Ricky was quite detached about his two sons; fond enough of them, I think, but uninvolved. On the other hand, he was very soppy about Sandie. There was one time when she came and stayed with us for ten days during the Easter holidays. I was very anxious that she'd be bored out of her head, and I arranged God knows what with every local activity I could think of, but the worst trouble I had turned out to be with Ricky crying his eyes out for two days after she went back to Ireland again. And yet it was only a couple of years later that he upped and left for Spanish domestic bliss with Madeleine. I think he was more or less out of touch with all of his offspring for quite a time after that, at his own choice. He had probably reinvented himself by then, and maybe the idea of being a father didn't really fit in with his new Spanish image."

"Hmmmm – parenthood for Narcissists! Now, that's an interesting one! For all my rummaging in the ol' text books, I still can't quite make out the parenthood bit with them." Alex flexed her elbows to and fro and then stretched her arms downwards as she considered this area of investigation. "It seems that generally, they like the idea of parenthood. There'll be a new orbit of power and control, this time over an adorable mini version of themselves. They can bask in reflected glory at having produced such a superb replica, and if, by any chance, there is a positive unusualness about the kids (like they're identical twins, for example) the additional attention on the product is felt as a reflection of their stupendous achievement.

"After all, whatever a baby is like, women tend to make adoring noises at it, don't they? I think a Narcissist male takes those noises as admiration of him, for producing such a fine specimen or two, and also because he believes the infants' delightfully attractive charm reminds the cooing audience of his own considerable adult ones. But as soon as the child is old enough to be an individual who challenges his authority or does not attract so much general admiration, a Narcissist tends to lose interest. He will, of course, very much resent the child if his partner focuses her attention on the kid rather than on him. Generally, I don't think many Narcissists handle parenthood very well in the long run."

"But they can appear to be amazingly attached to their kids, you know," Jenny observed. "And the staggering thing is how attached and loyal their kids seem to remain to them, despite selfish behaviour which must be blatantly obvious, even to their devoted progeny. I sometimes wonder if Narcissists may exhibit a flair for parenthood with young children because their own self absorption is very similar to the terrible two year old's. I know you'd think that two or more spoilt toddlers would squabble and compete, but that doesn't always happen, does it? I think that's because toddlers click that they can match one another as playmates.

"Maybe there is a subconscious recognition between our Narcissist as Developmentally Arrested Adult and a blithely self centred Child; they have a sort of peer group compatibility, despite the age difference. As I said, Joe was an excellent father to my two when they were very young. He seemed absolutely fascinated by the various stages of their development, which touched me very much. I thought his close observation of them as mini eco systems reflected a very special quality in him. To me, it meant he wasn't just a high principled eco warrior, talking the walk, but a devoted family man who cared about the planet from a profoundly personal, as well as humanitarian, perspective. He seemed to have an intuitive sense of playfulness with the children which was a delight to watch, and a total contrast to my own purposeful parenting. He was their hero, and his influence on them ran very deep.

"The trouble was, once he moved on to another family, and then a third, new arenas and women and step children would take his attention for a while, and his interest in his first pair of kids waned. It was the same with the planet, actually. After he set up home with Molly, he dropped all the ecological idealism and took to wearing Gucci shoes and Armani suits. The children told me that when they eventually got to visit their father and Molly in their new, white carpeted home, they were provided with a sparsely furnished spare room to sleep in, with no attempt to make it a space for children. Julie peered into a wardrobe, apparently, which was crammed full of all Joe's designer stuff, with no room left for the children's clothes or possessions. And this was the man who had remarked to me early in our break up, 'I think the children should come and live with me because Molly and I can be a proper family for them.'

"As time went on, although he established a routine of having the children one weekend every three weeks and for a week or two in alternate holidays, he really seemed pretty casual about giving them attention or opportunities to enjoy themselves. He appeared increasingly less connected with them as they grew older, and although he was still observant about them to some extent, he would tend to pinpoint Matt and Julie's vulnerabilities, and actually seemed to get pleasure out of playing on them. Maybe he did that as a way of getting me to acknowledge that the bad parent was me, not him? Is that projection, Alex? Trying to get me to take on what he feared about himself? Anyway, he used to tease Julie for her chubbiness and Matt for his dreaminess, but 'tease' isn't really the right word because I think the kids felt his criticisms in a way that scarred their hearts. Dreadful thought! To have given them a father who latterly set out to break their spirits and block their potential is a terrible burden to bear!"

Both women sighed in unison, although Jenny's expression bore the brunt of this demoralising lament; she pulled down the corners of her mouth in a grimace of remorse before continuing, "Julie still has a problem with food, and Matt seems to have been left with a deep rooted horror of unpleasantness. He has developed that act of affable passivity which means any negative comment or thought he encounters simply bounces off him without being registered. Couldn't you see that act of nonchalance in him this morning? If Joe hadn't bonded with both kids so brilliantly when they were very young, I think both of them would have been more able to cope with his negativity when it began to filter in later, during their early adolescence and beyond. As it was, the chasm between Joe's early intuitive intimacy and his later casual indifference was, I think, unendurable at some level.

"The sad thing is that although I know this, I can't find a way to talk to either of them about it. I wish I could get across to them that the change of attitude was never about *them* being lovable or not; it was about Joe's personal difficulties in sustaining love. Matt seems somehow to have shouldered full responsibility for his father and is, in effect, 'fathering' him! As for Julie, she is permanently hurt by her dad and relentlessly bitter. So this 'Love them/Leave them' aspect of their father's parenting probably won't ever be available to either of them for discussion. I suppose Joe must have felt loving towards them in his own way when they were very young, to have been so profoundly connected with them initially."

Jenny sighed, shrugging her shoulders slightly, attempting to relieve a slight stiffness in her neck.

" 'Love – whatever that means…' " Alex giggled at her inept attempt to misquote Prince Charles in his own particular mode of speech. She glanced out at the landscape, noticing with some alarm that they seemed to be climbing into remote terrain. Far ahead of them, the route they were taking snaked up through the moors and there was a misty bleakness about their surroundings which discomforted her. It was several seconds before Alex spoke again.

"I think that's maybe what we learn best from our dear Narcissists – what Love isn't. Maybe as a result of that, we come to understand a bit better what it is. Back to the idea that the personality is honed by its awareness of anti love, or whatever the wording of Scott Peck's line is. Anyway, perhaps we could write a sort of modern parallel to that passage from the Bible. You know, 'Love suffereth long and is kind …. endureth all things and never fails'; that list of what 'Love' is. Can't remember more than a smattering of it. Oh dear! I think it says what 'Love' isn't, as well…… 'is not puffed up, does not delight in evil….'

"We could probably do our own version, if we thought about it hard, making it helpful in sorting out what is real reciprocal Love and what is actually Narcissistic targeting and supplying. We were devoted suppliers, Jenny, sure enough. But never failing in our dedication to shore up our beloved Narcissists' psychological identities is not necessarily Love, is it? I know it certainly feels like we're loving them, but, if I force myself to face up to the truth, it's probably more about obsessive need to be needed, or addiction to bonding with an unavailable man, such as our fathers were to us. We need to look at where we were coming from before we got targeted."

"Hmpff," replied Jenny, shuddering momentarily. "Self analysis holds little appeal for me, I must say. Anyway, I think that biblical passage you're on about is from Corinthians. I had to learn a section of it somewhere back in the mists of time. There was something about not keeping a record of old wounds and never giving up on another person. If that's right, then, actually, we certainly wouldn't qualify for loving either of our Narcissists, would we? We spend countless hours reliving their sins with each other, after all! And we constantly attempt to smash any hope we have of regarding them as real, loving human beings. Perhaps we are just as bad as they are. That's an unnerving thought, isn't it?"

"No, it isn't," replied Alex firmly. "It isn't unnerving because we actually know it isn't true, Jenny. The reason we work at reliving their behaviours and smashing our hopes of them is not because we wish to delight in evil, or enjoy being nasty about them. It's because we are struggling to regain our own sanity. We do still love them obsessively; we probably always will, I'm afraid. But it isn't a healthy love for us because it involves us being subsumed by them. That isn't even relevant to what they want of us any longer, and there's no point whatsoever in us supplying something superfluous to their requirements. Ideally, we'd learn to hate the relationship dysfunction without any rejection of them, as people we happen to love. The trouble is, that's more or less impossible to achieve when their sense of Self has become so distorted by lethal defence strategies that we can't distinguish between their disorder and their personality.

"Anyway, don't you find that there's never any point in trying to use any one section of definitive scripture to inform our outlook on life because there'll be another part of the same source which will give a contradictory message? For example, Christ said, 'Love thy neighbour as thyself' which would indicate it's okay to love, or we might say rather, to take care of yourself. He didn't say 'not thyself.' So I could use that bit of the Bible to say, 'We must look after ourselves first, before we try to take care of others.' Or I could pick out, 'Charity begins at home,' or 'Cast ye the mote out of your own eye before you try to get the mote out of your mate's eye.' Any of that lot could back up an argument which refutes the idea of always putting the other person first. It's a bit dicey to claim that Love suffereth long and is perpetually credulous and kind. To hope eternally for mutual love when your head is being done in by exploitative pseudo love strikes me as downright daft. Yet that's exactly what I did, to my eternal shame."

"Look, this is Llangollen, coming up soon," interrupted Jenny, waving towards her right. "There's lots of good archaeological stuff round here including a very impressive hill site fort, and superb scenery. The Offa's Dyke walk is more than 150 miles. It really is a great trek with an amazing variety of landscapes to please any walker. It's smattered with lovely old towns in among woodlands and gorges and mountain ridges and valleys and hills but this is the only part that I know, really. It wasn't that far to come when my parents moved to live near Much Wenlock."

Alex nodded, attempting to look enthused by the delights of the area. She hoped that there would soon be further comforting signs of civilisation, but did not want to communicate this thought. Jenny meanwhile wound back the most recent sentences of their conversation in her mind and returned to the interchange.

"I've never understood what on earth that phrase means in practice – 'Love Yourself', she commented. "How can we possibly do that and not be a Narcissist? That's what *they* do!"

"Back to our questions about whatever 'Love is', or isn't." Alex shifted slightly in the seat, as if, in so doing, she was stating her position more conclusively. "If we think 'Love' means letting the other person get away with whatever they want and indulging them unconditionally at our own expense, that doesn't work very well when we apply it to ourselves, does it? It means – um – well, we eat as much chocolate as we want and get very unfit and immobile, and probably don't have many friends because they get pissed off with us indulging ourselves all the time and never listening to the other person's point of view. However, think of that Baltimore church thing of the Sixties: 'Beyond a wholesome discipline, be kind to yourself; you too are a child of the universe.... you have a right to be here. Strive to be happy...' I think that's more along the right lines."

"*Strive* to be happy?" echoed Jenny. "Surely we can't work at happiness? It's a contradiction in terms."

"Hmmm, I agree it's an odd phrase. I think that part of it could be said better. 'Strive to create the conditions around you which are likely to promote your own happiness' might be more appropriate, but it's an awful mouthful! I do think it is accurate enough though, as a pointer to what loving ourselves means. So often we think we need unwholesome discipline, and we kick ourselves, and act as if we don't deserve any sort of contentment. We might actually set out to be of life saving service to others' hearts and minds, without pausing for one moment to consider whether that quest is likely to be genuinely effective, either for ourselves or for the unfortunate recipients of our efforts.

"It seems to be some sort of martyr complex in us, to seek suffering and then dignify it with the status of self sacrifice. Is that the inheritance of a Western culture based on distorted Christian ideals? I think that I put up with damaging treatment from both Liam and Marcus without protest, imagining it was compassionate towards them and character building for me to behave like that. What crap! You might say that the philosophy behind it is that the person you love must be fervently encouraged to recognise his child of the universe status, even to the detriment of your own state of being. How could that be a healthy attitude to encourage in him? And it certainly didn't do me much good either!

"Perhaps we both thought that's how it worked, Jenny, because of how our mums subtly coaxed our dads, encouraging them by modelling consistent resilience and determination. Helped by their wives, both men overcame real social disadvantage to become rapidly upwardly mobile, even back in the Forties and Fifties, when the class boundaries must have still been firmly in place. All four of our men, in the next generation, originally wanted to be upwardly mobile too, and might surely have expected an easier time of it in the late Sixties, than our fathers' generation before them. I suppose it'd be true to say that of the four of the men we chose, only Marcus actually acquired a sustained higher level of social status in the end. That must be the world of academia for you; once you've gained your place, it's probably quite difficult to tumble out of the realms of intellectual elitism.

"But I'm waffling again – sorry! Our mums – um, yes! My dear ol' mum, just like yours, had a hold over her three kids' lives which Dad let her exercise because he didn't seem to want it. So she knew more about us than he ever could. That meant increasing power to her as we kids grew nearer to being adults. Once we got to be over sixteen, Mum began to enjoy our company more, and valued our conversation – well, Bryan's and mine, anyway.

"She actually used the power of that close mother/teenager relationship she had, to our considerable benefit. A good example was her managing to persuade my father to let Bryan marry Liz while they were both still at university. Dad was set against it because he felt a man shouldn't marry until he had an income. As it turned out, their student marriage gave Bryan a year and a half of happy domesticity with Liz before he was killed climbing Mont Blanc. It made a lot of difference to Liz, heartbroken though she was, that she had had that time living with him, and that she was left his widow, not just an unlucky girlfriend."

Alex paused. The landscape around them was looking even bleaker now.

"Er – is that where we're heading?" She waved in the direction of the distant mountain road.

"Yes. Eerie, isn't it? Somewhere near here there's a place called 'World's End' and it's easy to see why! But then lots of places are called 'World's End'. I suppose it depends on how big or small the person's world was, if you get me. Um ... I wanted to make a point then about our mums – what was it?" Jenny frowned with the effort of retrieving her train of thought, and then re boarded it triumphantly. "Yes! You forget, Alex; both our mums had another big advantage over us – their husbands didn't leave them! The pairings both stayed intact, however much the actual bond relied on collusion and uneven distribution of public status and recognition. Our fathers were surely better husbands at some level than Joe or Liam? They were more committed to the family life they had signed up for."

"I'm not sure whether we can say that they were better men," mused Alex. "I think they probably had parallel difficulties to those Joe and Liam endured as children and adolescents. I would have thought the psychological damage was quite similar in that little quartet – our two fathers and our two young husbands. Girls marry their fathers, remember! Maybe the difference is that both your dad and mine were in rather a mess emotionally but they could sometimes be gently coaxed into revealing bits of their vulnerability in private to their trusted spouses. It would appear that Joe and Liam had been so profoundly threatened psychologically that they closed down their access to their own vulnerability. This would make it inevitable that they couldn't have empathy for anyone else either, particularly not for someone in intimate connection with them.

"Either Joe or Liam could, of course, feel intense emotion if the act they had created as an image of perfection was undermined in any way, and could even weep about it. But I would say that they were weeping for a construction rather than mourning the loss of something deep at the heart of them.

"As far as I can see, Narcissists don't actually mourn Loss; it's far too awful for them to go there. They've lost out on Selfhood since their infancy and that makes Loss so all-encompassing that it would utterly destroy them to register it fully. That's why, unlike our dads, Joe and Liam could sail abruptly out of a marriage, even with two small kids and a relatively benign relationship with their wife. They had cut off their own deepest feelings of connection with anyone else, out of self protection, and thus had no access to those responses when they abandoned one family set up for another. They can't actually feel at the deepest level. I don't think they can register a negative emotion which reaches down beyond anger in some form or another. That condition is simultaneously their greatest protection and their most devastating deficiency.

"I think sometimes they sense their shallowness of feeling, and that means they seek to pick up the trappings of sincere emotional interchanges from others. Marcus used to talk about 'deep and meaningfuls' with some amusement, as a label for a communicative conversation; as if it was a game he had to play along with, sometimes. After all, if you or I lost a leg, we'd probably be fitted out with an artificial one, wear trousers a lot, and try to walk as if we had a normal pair of pins. We might even forget at times that we were disguising our one leggedness. Isn't it human nature to seek to mask our shortcomings? It seems that nowadays, we find falsity quite acceptable in relation to the physical body – false leg, false boobs, face lift, hair extensions and so on. But we regard it as hideous deception if it involves simulation of empathy and connectedness.

"Maybe Narcissists forget that they can't feel because they've long accustomed themselves to acting as if they can, to the extent that other people generally accept their act as real. So Narcissists may not have the faintest idea that they're being false in their intimate relationships. It must be very confusing not to have your gut feelings there as indicators for how you might authentically connect with others."

"Well, I can certainly see the attractions of not being able to feel," remarked Jenny, with a half smile.

"It's not that great, I suspect," mused Alex, eyes screwed up. She was observing from the distant lie of the land ahead that they would be descending towards lower terrain soon, and felt cheered by this, as she expanded on her thought. "It must surely feel isolating, even if our Narcissists can't work out the whys and wherefores. Maybe the intensity of excitement when they find a new target person stimulates them wonderfully, and they experience it as Coming Alive Again. Perhaps they think that is due to some magical quality in the new target, but really, it's just about a new version of their image as 'lover and beloved' which they can now start to create for themselves all over again. Of course, it's actually built on foundations just as sandy as the last image-construction was. So, inevitably, they are doomed to repeat the same mistake over and over again. Doesn't strike me as much fun, at the end of the day." Alex was quoting from the composite information stored in her head, but there was a note of genuine concern in her voice. Jenny seemed irritated by the tone, and responded with some alacrity.

"But at least Narcissists still have bright new dawns, Alex. They retain Hope! We've lost that, haven't we? We are bereft of Faith, Hope and Charity, by the look of it. I have absolutely no faith left in any possibility of romantic relationships, as far as I'm concerned. I certainly don't feel charitable towards either Joe or Ricky. And though at some level, I suppose I must still love Ricky (if that's really what 'charity' means in modern parlance), I am doing everything I can to separate that feeling from anything even remotely associated with him. They, on the other hand, move into a new relationship of mutual adoration, full of faith and hope that this new 'Love' will be transformative.

"I ask you, who sounds happier – them or us? And even if it all goes pear-shaped for them, they will already have groomed a replacement to be waiting in the wings, and then the whole exciting Hope thing starts all over again. They don't dwell on what they've lost. There is a determined optimism about them which sends them forever forward to pastures new. I so admire that optimism and resilience! They don't learn from experience which means that past disasters don't have a sobering impact on their present relationships. I agree with you, I don't think they can feel profound pain at all, whereas I'm absolutely certain they can be all lit up with pleasure and sparkling anticipation. You can see why they don't want to seek help or have therapy; they've got it made for themselves! It's us other poor sods who are discarded along the wayside who fill the consultation rooms, not them. All the years we choose to spend in any sort of relationship is simply a Waste; nothing more or less. We waste our lives living with them or talking about them or trying to understand them. We'd be better off talking about the uses of potpourri."

"Oh, Jenny! Do you really think that?" Alex glanced across in consternation.

"Sometimes! But not actually on this journey. I do need your waffling to keep me awake. Don't worry, Alex. I doubt that either of us could sustain any sort of Domestic Goddess conversation for more than ten minutes anyway, whereas Relationship Dysfunction could keep you going for days! But actually, we're approaching terra incognita now. So grab your glasses and see if you can pick up the suggested route on the left hand page there..." Jenny jabbed at the appropriate sector of the open road atlas with her left hand.

"Right!"

"Our destination is within our grasp!" announced Jenny with mock pomposity, and for a brief moment, both women found themselves equally focused on the last stage of the journey as they headed down into Ruthin.

CHAPTER 7

Deepest Wales

Once they were out in open country again, Alex soon found herself wondering what distraction to offer next. She sensed Jenny was tiring of the current topic of conversation and she even felt a bit exhausted by it herself. The traffic was very light now and there was quite a way to go before precise directions would be required. It occurred to her that Jenny might like to return to her unfinished account of life with Joe and, after Alex's repeated request for her to do so, and a half-hearted protest about the dullness of the story and the inevitable element of repetition, Jenny seemed happy enough to take up her tale once more.

"Well… we got back to England, but we didn't find it easy to get a roof over our heads because it was quite a disadvantage me being obviously pregnant. Most flats or rooms said things like, 'No dogs, no children.' In the end we found somewhere grotty, and I got myself a job temping, working for an agency. I had to call on some very rusty typing and shorthand skills. I went for a job as an audio typist and when I first went working there, I told the personnel manager in the office that I happened not to have encountered this particular machine before. He very kindly explained the sort of audio dictaphone thing to me. I was supposed to type his letters for him after he had spoken them into this machine. I made so many mistakes that I had to hide away all my bogged up attempts and smuggle them home to destroy them, to make sure that no one realised how terrible I was! I gradually got better but then I had to move into other jobs which came up through the agency.

"I did a lot of envelope stuffing jobs which was boring beyond belief, and I also worked in a café at night to earn extra money. I waitressed up until a fortnight before Julie was born, negotiating my bump between the tables, but luckily it didn't show too much because I was pretty fit back then. The last job I had was working as a secretary at S.E. laboratories where they used me as a guinea pig to help develop the foetal heart monitor. Unfortunately, the scientist who was using me hadn't finished working on it when Julie arrived, so one of the engineers' wives took over my role. That was really quite interesting, you know. Actually, I did get a letter which was a thank you to 'Pip and her mother', but I don't know where it is – I've lost it! That's a shame really, because it would be nice for Julie to have it now. Whenever I see foetal heart monitors being used I think, 'Hmmm, yes; I remember all that.' I used to have to go in every day and be wired up for him to practise on. It never occurred to me that it might do any damage, but anyway, I'm sure it didn't." Jenny shrugged slightly, glancing across at Alex with a grin.

"Quite a claim to fame, you know," Alex commented in response. "What a medical pioneer you were! I'm very impressed!" She was yet again surprised by the variety of Jenny's life experience.

"Well, before Julie was born, we found a flat through friends of ours, which was the top floor of a three story house. We had a bit of a job persuading the people renting it to us that noise wouldn't carry down, but we arranged to put Julie's cot in the attic room inside a large cupboard space, and that seemed to do the trick. So it was a bed sitter and a kitchen and a bathroom which we shared with all the people downstairs. Joe had a collection of lizards and toads and snakes and things which we stacked in aquariums all up the wall in the kitchen and we lived with that. We painted the room purple and we were a couple of sort of self contained hippies, I suppose!

"I produced Julie easily enough at Chiswick Maternity Home. It was well equipped and modern, and it was also a very efficient teaching hospital where I was extremely well looked after for ten blissful days. The only disadvantage was that I hadn't a clue what to do with this baby of mine, though I turned out to be an excellent cow, and there were several other babies in the hospital who were fed with my expressed milk.

"My mother came down to see me for a few days and she was a great help to me because I was absolutely terrified of this little bundle of a daughter. It was really hard because Julie didn't thrive as she should at first, and she was very tiny anyway. It seemed to be because she would drink too much of my copious milk too quickly and then bring it straight up again. I was totally unskilled as a mother and there wasn't the support then that there is nowadays. There was a health visitor but I remember she was very airy fairy, and they certainly didn't keep an eye on you, as they do now. And then, blow me down! Julie was three months old and I found out I was pregnant again which was quite a shock, I can tell you!

"They said back then that if you were breast feeding you couldn't get pregnant, but I can definitely let you know that that's an old wives' tale! I felt as if I was pregnant for about two years because one pregnancy led into the next so rapidly. But there are, of course, some benefits in having two children so close together. They were more like twins, and that means that you get through the developmental stages so much quicker. But once Matt was born, I have to say that it was absolutely exhausting. I felt as if I was in a fog of tiredness for his first six months, but then that's the same for any young mother really, and I was a lot fitter then, back in my youth. I had a great deal more energy, too.

"Anyway, we lived in this little flat, and I joined forces with an architect's wife and she designed little mob caps and dungarees which I had to sew. They were ever so trendy and brightly coloured, and exactly the sort of cotton numbers that your early Seventies children would wear. It took a long time to take off, this business, but I also had sewing – making aprons – which was a bloody awful job. I had got outreach work which meant I went and collected a whole pile of bits of material, brought them home, sewed them all up and then took the finished articles back. We were paid peanuts for it, absolute peanuts, and I had to use all my own electricity. I think that outreach sewing just about paid the milk bill every week, and I was working extremely hard.

"One day, I went back to this man and said to him, 'Well – you know – this is ridiculous, working for peanuts.' And he just said to me – I'll never forget it – he said, 'You don't want the work, love?

There's hundreds that do out there!' So I paused for a moment and then I said, 'No, I don't want the work. I'm not going to do this!' And luckily, as the architect's wife's sewing stuff was doing rather well, I was able to drop the apron work.

"Meanwhile, Joe had returned to managing a pet shop which he had been doing before we went to Africa. I had so wanted him to go back to college but that was not to be. I remember a walk we took in Richmond Park around that time. We were having this discussion about what to do with our future. We were both very young, of course; he was twenty, I think, and I was twenty one. I could see that it was time we accepted a certain level of responsibility, introduced a career into the picture and sort of 'grew up'. He told me that there was no way that I could support the family while he took up studying. His take on it back then was that he could earn much more than I could. Therefore, what on earth was the point of doing it the other way round? I realise now that, in fact, he was using me as an excuse, and that he didn't actually have the nerve to go back to college.

"There were grants available back then, and I knew perfectly well that we could have pulled together and got through it with me being the main wage earner. I wasn't particularly happy about his decision. The only thing is that I knew he was the one who had to make the choice. If I'd insisted on doing it my way and it all went pear-shaped later, he would blame me. But I was very disappointed about it.

"Anyway, as I've said, my grandmother had died. I hadn't been to the funeral because my mother hadn't wanted me to go, just after Julie's birth. It was soon afterwards that my mother decided to help us out financially, as I told you. My aunt and uncle also had some money to invest because they had inherited money through my grandmother as well. They decided that they would buy a big property, and I think part of my aunt's motive was to use some of her inheritance from her mother's will to help me, as she had always felt rather sorry for me. My uncle Paul, however, was a business man, and he decided he would use this money from his mother-in-law to buy the building, but he was prepared to set Joe and myself up in business in the process. So they would be coming into business with us.

"Well, Joe had the pet shop. I had wanted him to go back to university and study Zoology but he had refused to go down that avenue on the pretext that I couldn't earn enough to keep him, as I've said. He was dead right, of course, but it depends what you mean by 'enough'. I do remember thinking that things would be so much better if he did get a degree, and I was sure we could scrape by. It didn't seem to matter to me if we had to scrimp for two or three years, if the end result was that he could get a much better job and feel good that he had achieved things academically. He was certainly bright enough to go but I do think it was a confidence thing really.

"So Joe decided to go into business, and Paul bought this building in their village and that's how The Water Life Centre came into being. We moved from the little Teddington flat with all the reptiles up against the kitchen wall, with baby Julie, and with Matt soon to arrive in December. We had actually been told by our Teddington landlords that we had to vacate the flat because it consisted of just two rooms and they weren't prepared to have two kids living there. They had only just tolerated Julie because she slept stuffed in the semi soundproof cupboard. So we had to get out and we went to stay with my aunt and uncle for about three months, I think, in their lovely house in Ferndown.

"Matt was born in Guildford hospital. I was very well looked after and I had no worries about my eventual departure from the ward because I had my aunt (Mum's sister) as an extremely efficient supportive carer from the moment of his arrival. Of course, my dear mother came down from Much Wenlock to stay with my aunt and uncle, and to take charge of Julie.

"Once Matt and I arrived back from the hospital, I was kept in bed, I remember, and this baby was brought into me for feeding and then promptly removed by one or other of the sisters. Otherwise, I was free to indulge myself during the day in somewhat isolated luxury! Joe and Paul were hard at work every day which meant I was very much under the control of these two women. Oh, and then they invited Joe's mother over to meet The Baby. My mother certainly went into nurse mode when their guest arrived. Eileen was presented with afternoon tea in a very formal way and, bless her, she coped with these two officious sisters very well. Apparently, she was then permitted to receive this baby into an appropriate embrace. I was marooned in bed upstairs – and, you know, she was told she could hold her new grandson.

"Obviously, I suppose they made polite conversation for a while and Eileen was allowed to go on holding her grandson, and I presume they were still sipping tea and looking at this baby when my mother must have said, 'Right, that's enough!' and taken him away. Oh dear! I'm so glad I wasn't downstairs to see that. Anyway, dear Eileen survived it all successfully, and told me about it later, with considerable amusement!

"Well, within a couple of months, we could move into the flat above the shop and Joe was able to start trading as The Water Life Centre. He was a very hard worker and knew his stuff, and he was also a very good salesman; he could sell absolutely anything to anybody, actually. The business took off, and worked well for quite a while. He got a considerable reputation and people came to him from all around the place. He became specialised in salt water fish – you know – salt water tanks. He actually got involved with one of the James Bond films and was seconded out for a bit, to work on the set. He really did work extremely hard, and business was flourishing. This was back in '71 – '72. But then, of course, there was a recession and – er – also, along with the recession, there was the horrid realisation that how people were collecting these marine fish and animals was not really ecologically sound, by any means. I feel a bit guilty now but, of course, we didn't know. However, ignorance isn't really a valid excuse, is it?

"So things were going wrong, and we decided we needed to shut down the business before it actually went under. It was obvious to us all that we had to close it down, and we were in '74 or '75 by now which meant times were hard. However, Joe quickly found another job as a salesman, through a friend in the village. As I said, he could sell an Arab a raincoat in the desert; he was that sort of a salesman. It was all Thai imported goods, carvings, wind chimes, that sort of thing, because the guy in the village was married to a Thai girl.

"After a while, though, another friend, Jez Elliot, offered Joe a chance to work for him. He had a photographic developing business and at first, Joe was a sort of sales rep but eventually he was given a shop or two to manage. It was around then that he met the teenage model, Molly. He and Jez used to go to lunch at the pub near the Reading shop. She used to drop into the pub for her lunch break too, from her work. The first I knew about it was when Joe began saying that he had met this girl; that for the first time he had met somebody who he could actually get on with! I'd ask, 'What did you do at lunch time today, darling?' And he'd reply, 'Oh, well, we went to the pub, and there was a really nice crowd there and there was this one girl and I could really talk to her....' And as soon as he said that, I remember that I felt the hairs go up on the back of my neck. I knew I'd never heard him speak about anyone like that before.

"At the same time, Uncle Paul was getting rid of the building and once the business had been sold, we had to move out pretty quickly. We found a flat above a garage just down the road from where we had been living, and we walked down the pavement with all our belongings on our backs, in countless relay operations. We were told we could live there for six weeks but we ended up staying there for six months. It was a horrid, damp flat. We had a 'put you up' in the sitting room. The children had the bedroom with their bunk beds in the middle of the room because there was mould all over the walls and it was a terribly cold winter. But, you know what? It was the only time that both children were extremely well all winter! They were away from the central heating in the flat we'd had in Paul's building, and that made me very conscious of the need to keep them warm whenever we were at home. I was extra careful that they were well dressed in pyjamas and dressing gowns and things, and snuggled up after a hot bath at night; lots of blankets and that sort of thing.

"I remember that around about then, Joe had sort of 'gone away with the fairies'. He seemed to be in total denial about the state we were living in. By now, I had a job at an art gallery. I had spent four years or so helping to run Joe's business, doing all the books, and I also had a part time job helping at a play group where I was the treasurer, and did some general admin work, too. But I felt I was getting bored and isolated. You know how it is, Alex, with two young kids. Once Matt was four and a half, I applied for a part time job working in the gallery and I got it!

"I used to cycle to work, and the job was for two and a half hours, five days a week. Even though it didn't pay well, it was a very good job for me. I had, after all, been to art school for a while, and I had enough business experience to deal with any of the gallery's transactions which came my way. I was the assistant exhibitions officer. I remember when I was being interviewed, Hester asked me who my favourite artist was and I replied that the one I didn't like was Cezanne. She asked me why I didn't like him and I gave some senseless reason why. Actually, my dislike was based on the fact that my art college tutor way back had liked him and I had loathed her! Anyway, Hester was a bit eccentric, and I guess my answers seemed normal enough to her, and she reckoned I could do the job! So I got it.

"I must admit, it really was a lovely job and I thoroughly enjoyed it. I had to work every other Saturday but the children could come, too. They could sit in the little restaurant place and they would position themselves there and count people in. They had a clicker to do the counting and they loved that. In the holidays, there would be workshops in the library which was at the back of the gallery, or in the museum which had an adult education room in it. And I used to say to the children, 'You've got to go to this workshop. You'll be read to all morning – and you will do it.' And they just used to go along and attend these courses.

"But anyway, we had come out of the pet shop business with just about enough money to put down a deposit on a house. We were looking for a house in the area, and it was back in '78, when property prices were just beginning to rise after a long slump. We found this place in Liphook – 19, Woodside Lane – and we went down to see it. It was a semi-detached, very ordinary council type property, but it had three bedrooms and it was in a cul de sac. But the best thing was that it backed onto wooded land and a little stream. I just thought of the children; I knew it would be a nice place for them. We bought it on a mortgage of £12,500, which was a big burden for us. But we moved in and John's brother helped with his minivan, bless him. Buying that house was the best thing I ever did."

Alex nodded and murmured, 'God, yes!', thinking of her own good luck, made possible by a generous loan from her parents, to be able to buy a very cheap London flat in the early '80s, during an on-going slump in the market there. That flat had been a godsend to her, too, as she had started to rebuild a life for herself and her sons after Liam's departure. It was easy to appreciate the vital importance of Jenny's bricks and mortar, knowing roughly how the story was to unfold. She glanced across at Jenny, wondering if approaching the most painful part of the narrative would be difficult to combine with the demands of driving, but Jenny's posture seemed free from tension, her hands loosely holding the steering wheel, brow smooth. Her tone was equally relaxed as she carried on speaking.

"Joe was going backwards and forwards to Reading, of course, still doing the photography job, and I'd got myself a moped to carry on with the gallery job in Guildford. Joe had the use of a car for his job which was sort of on loan to him. We obviously couldn't afford to buy one ourselves. Moped traveling wasn't that great. I had two accidents in eighteen months, and neither of them was my fault! But it was living a bit out of town that had made our house affordable, since it was cheaper to live over the border in Hampshire than in Surrey, back then. It was just right for the kids! There were all these other children to play with in the street, and they could go round the back and along the stream, running wild. They hated their new school, of course, and with reason, because it was a lousy school.

"We had moved in the April when the kids were about eight and seven. Between September and December, various strange things started to happen. Joe began to lose an awful lot of weight. I kept finding these long blonde hairs on his jumper. He kept staying away from home, which he had been doing before for his travelling sales stuff, but now it was becoming more frequent. He said he was often staying with his friend, Tony, and I accepted that, but I was uneasy about it all.

"Finally, we got to December. It was Boxing Day, actually. We went out for a pub meal and I suppose I must have been boosted somehow by a glass of wine because I suddenly said, 'Look here, we've got to sort things out. What has been going wrong?' And he said, 'Well, what do you think?' So I said, 'No, for me, there isn't anything wrong. We've been through the sale of the business and the building; we've got a house now and we're just beginning to get ourselves a bit of security. But, all the same, I feel there is something wrong.' Joe just said there was nothing wrong for him, either.

"Well, two days later I rang up Joe's friend, Tony, the one who Joe said he'd been staying with on and off during the last four months. I asked him what he thought was wrong with Joe and I explained that I couldn't get through to him at all. I said, 'Somehow we seem unable to discuss anything. I've asked him if there's another woman, and I don't think there is, but as he's been coming and staying with you, I wondered if you've been able to talk to him?' And Tony just said, 'I haven't seen Joe in months.'

"So then I went back and questioned Joe. He finally told me more about his relationship with Molly. And I said that we'd been through so much! Surely he didn't want a divorce? He waffled around and said he didn't know what he wanted. So from January until March I did everything I could possibly think of to make it work, which included jumping on him sexually whenever I got the opportunity! I had decided that he couldn't possibly keep playing away if he was more than satisfied at home. So whenever I saw him, I hit on him and oh, he must have thought his ship had come in! Both of us ended up losing a lot more weight, actually. I just pretended that nothing was wrong, and worked very hard at the idea of keeping the family happy and together and all that. Outwardly, I was being nice and not showing any anger. After all, I could easily understand that he was attracted to a nineteen year old model who probably worshipped him.

"What I did find very hard was that over quite a while he had started to be very nasty to me with words; this was actually well before he met Molly. He had begun to – er – turn, and he used to put me down an awful lot. But I used to think, 'Well, that's just him! He loves me, really; it's just his way of showing me affection, in a roundabout sort of style.' After all, we were still very active sexually, and I would have thought that sex would have been the first thing to go! If you don't desire the other person, then obviously, it's pretty likely that it's all over, but there still seemed to be plenty of desire.

"My mother used to drive all the way down from Much Wenlock and visit us occasionally, especially while we were still in that grotty flat, and she was worried about the way Joe spoke to me back then, I remember. She would bring food parcels – Red Cross parcels, really! – and she'd always bring a bit of beef and my children would exclaim, 'Granny! Meat!' I'd been feeding them on beans and fish heads and stuff because, you know, we didn't have any money.

"I remember once when we were still in the flat, my mother had said, 'You two ought to go out to the pub; I'll look after the children.' So I went up and put on something clean and tidy. I remember that I came back down, and she turned to Joe and said to him, 'Oh, doesn't Jenny look lovely!' And Joe just dismissed it without a word, and turned away. I felt very hurt at that. Anyway, once we were living in the house we'd just bought and we were really going at it sexually, I think he did sort of try to put things back together with me. He told me that he had changed pubs and he was trying not to see Molly any more.

"I didn't question him about whether he was still in touch with her because I wanted it all to feel good to him at home. I had secretly been thinking of going along and seeing her parents and telling them about it, but then one night we seemed to conclude that our marriage was worth saving, and he wanted to keep with the children and anyway, think of the consequences of what he was doing; we could get through this together, as I saw it.

"He was still away some nights but I never questioned him because I thought nagging about it was the way to lose him altogether. I was very understanding, I suppose, but it just seemed the most sensible way to behave, in the circumstances. With all the wisdom of my twenty nine years, I was under the impression that given the right sort of space, he would come through this as just a temporary hiatus time which eventually we would put behind us.

"He had told me that he had been finding life very difficult with me over the last few years. I don't know whether he had actually said he didn't love me anymore. (Did he have any idea of what 'Love' was, though?) He certainly implied that life with me was not what it had been. But I had pointed out to him that the initial passion and love between two people will change over nine years and with two children, especially with reversals of fortune and disappointed career hopes, yet we were still bonking like nobody's business, so surely we could get through the hard times we had had?

"By this time, though, I was down to skin and bone. I think I had lost a couple of stone in weight. We got to the end of February, and one Friday, Joe was going away on a karate weekend. I was relieved when he went on these jaunts because I thought, 'Oh, well! At least he's getting rid of his frustrations!' But he said he needed the car, and it was a weekend that I was working at the gallery next day, and it would be very hard for me to organise my Saturday if I hadn't got transport to bring the children with me to work. To have the car would have been very useful to me. But I remember he made every possible excuse for being in urgent need of the car himself which meant that I would have to resort to using the moped. I obviously must have had to ferry the children somewhere before I went to work; I can't remember now what I did. But anyway, I remember thinking, 'He's still seeing her.'

"I knew then that this had gone on long enough. I went to see a solicitor that Friday afternoon, and I said, 'Look, my husband is seeing another woman. I don't want to instigate a divorce. We have two children, and we've had a good life together. What can I do?' He was a very nice guy, the solicitor; young, sympathetic. (I heard that he subsequently died in a car accident, poor bloke) Anyway, he said, 'Well, I will write a letter and it will say all of this. But it will also indicate that the affair has got to stop.'

So I said, 'Fine, thank you. ' Back home I came, feeling a lot better! The following day, the letter arrived through the post, with the solicitor's office stamp on the envelope, addressed to Joe. So I put it on the mantelpiece to await Joe's return from the karate weekend. I had been planning to confront the guilty couple at the hotel but I had decided not to. What was the point? What would I do to myself? It would just make a fool of somebody and that somebody was obviously going to be me. So I didn't do that.

"Joe came home from the weekend and subsequently saw the letter up on the mantelpiece. I remember the moment so clearly. He picked it up, read it, turned round and walked out without a word. He went and stayed in a B and B. I had no idea where he was going. He then rang me up and asked me what I wanted. I said that I didn't know but did he want a divorce? He said, 'Yes'. And then he said, 'I'll arrange it all so that you don't have to sue me for divorce.' He meant that he would acknowledge he had committed adultery with an unknown party; I think that was how you could get the most rapid divorce back then. He settled into the B and B, presumably with Molly. But then, I remember he kept ringing me up saying things like, Could he have the calor gas fire? He was a bit cold. And then it would be, Could he have X Y and Z? Because, you know, he didn't have them there. And I said, 'No!' I thought he could just get on with whatever it was he had chosen to do.

"Shortly after that, he and Molly moved into a house together. I had said to the children, 'It's nothing to do with you – it's to do with me ….. Daddy doesn't love me anymore and doesn't want to be here with me. He still loves you two and that's that.'

"Julie was beside herself; she was absolutely hysterical. She was just nine years old by now, and Matt was eight – he dealt with it by blanking it all out. I rang Joe and said to him, 'You need to come and talk to your daughter and reassure her that you love her.' So he came and he did, and he spoke to both of them. He talked to them for some time, and it worked because actually, the only thing that was going to change in their lives was that their father was no longer in the house. They saw and heard almost nothing of him for a few months, but otherwise, their world held fairly steady. Friends down the road were there as ever, and Nanny and Granddad were still living quite near and in close touch. This was Joe's parents and they had been told, and were very upset about it. I think poor Eileen felt very guilty about what had happened. They were as supportive as they could possibly be, and they used to come down every Sunday to help in any way they could. When I eventually began to feel a bit better, I had to almost wean them off me! They were utterly dedicated to helping out in every practical aspect of our lives.

"My father wrote to Joe, a very nice letter, asking him why this had happened. Although he and Joe hadn't got on at all well when we had first met and got married, my father had come to realise what a successful relationship Joe had appeared to have with me, and what a good father he was to our children. Joe replied to the letter and said that the reason why he had fallen out of love with me was that I had let myself go. That was the reason. My mother told me all this later, I think. Certainly, I must have looked pretty gaunt.

"That was March 13th, when Joe left. In May half term week, I remember that Julie was due to go off to Guide and Brownie Camp.

I've told you this bit already, Alex!"

"Not properly. Go on!" replied Alex immediately.

"Well, er – I was still working in the gallery of course, which meant I needed both children to be catered for during that week. Anyway, Julie was complaining of stomach upsets and she used to be a bit apt to moan about being unwell. So I just ignored it and sent her off for an activity course during that week. Then, at the camp, she started being sick. Apparently, she went riding and could barely keep on the back of the pony! She was sent back home, and she was just lying on the sofa. I rang my mother and she said, 'Well, look; if it's still the same tomorrow,' – it was a Saturday – 'you must get in touch with an emergency doctor.' So the next morning, I rang the doctor but there was something wrong with the line and I couldn't get through to the weekend service. One of my friends from down the road came over. She was married to an ambulance driver, and she took one look at Julie and said to me that I simply must get hold of an ambulance. I said that I couldn't do that because Julie only had enteritis or something, but my friend insisted, and it was actually she who dialled 999.

"The ambulance duly turned up with flashing blue lights. Julie's hands by this time were cramped up because of lack of oxygen. I left Matt with friends and got into the ambulance with her and we sped to the hospital. Obviously, my friend's description of Julie's condition over the phone must have been spot on. When he had arrived at our house and laid eyes on Julie, the ambulance driver had immediately confirmed that it looked like acute appendicitis and phoned through to the hospital. They were all ready and waiting for her in the operating theatre when we were rushed through Emergency, but even so, her appendix burst when she was on the operating table. They were able to deal with it and put a drain in and stuff, but it was a very close run thing.

"So, of course, my mother came down, along with my father, I think, on yet another mercy mission. She was keen to take over the nursing of Julie because she didn't consider the hospital good enough. Joe did come to visit Julie but I don't know much about that because obviously, I had to be with Matt at home, or going back and forth between the two children. My mother was actually horrified by what she considered to be insufficient care and cleanliness standards in the hospital. There were cracked tiles and that sort of thing; they were building a new hospital at the time. She took one look at all this and declared, 'This is disgusting!' The sister on the ward said, 'Well, I'm sorry but we can't discharge this girl because the district nurses are on strike just now, and she needs nursing.' So my mother drew herself to her full height and announced, 'I am a nurse. I will look after her; I will take full responsibility!' I was hiding behind my mother, feeling very embarrassed, of course. Anyway, that's what we did! We bundled Julie up and took her away, and my mother nursed her at home for a few weeks.

"There's photo of us all at around that time. We went down to Boscombe Harbour and I think my father must have taken it. And there is this picture of me with a shock of hair and a very thin face. I was terribly scrawny and I was wearing this scarf wrapped round and round my neck because I was like a Belsen survivor or something. It wasn't that long afterwards – probably May – that I was seriously suicidal and began plotting to do myself in with the carbon monoxide piped back into the interior of my car. I used to wake up at three o'clock every morning and go and sit on the loo and think to myself, 'I'm obviously bog ugly and nobody loves me; what future is there for me? So I might as well end it.' I did have a car because I had been given the loan of a Nissan Cherry for six weeks by Jez, who felt sorry for me, I expect. I kept delaying returning it, because it was so useful.

"Anyway, as I've said, the only thing that stopped me actually committing suicide was that I didn't want the children to be the ones to find me dead. It was logistically very difficult to arrange things so that the kids wouldn't be looking for me in alarm but also so that my friends, alerted to a potential need to step in suddenly for the kids, would have had no reason to guess I was up to something. So I suppose that was it! I had reached rock bottom and there was now nowhere to go but up. When I realised this, I said to myself, 'Oh well, I've just got to get on with it,' and there was really no other choice. Two of my friends who were art teachers were suggesting to me that I should train to be an art teacher, too. The school hours and holidays would mean I'd be able to look after my children and all that. My friends were saying to me, 'Look, if we can do it, so can you, Jenny!'

So I applied to study for an art teacher's degree in the May, and I got in for that September, with a very generous grant, which you could get, back in those good old days.

"And that was the overall saving of everything because in September, Joe started making noises about coming back. By this time, I'd got something new to aim for. And now I was able to feel angry with him, and cross about how things had ended up with him. Up until then, I felt I had to seem cooperative and nice enough to him for the kids' sake. I think I wanted his access to them to seem smooth and relaxed, from their point of view. I must admit it was good for morale that he was sniffing around again – he was still with Molly, of course – but I was beginning to get a sense of finding my Self, and it felt good. I didn't want to go backwards again and to be pulled back into feeling so bad about myself ever again. Maybe I was beginning to learn that I could decide how I felt about my life and my future. I might not be climbing a ladder yet, but at least I standing very close to the bottom rung, and I was looking upwards!

"So there we are! Now it's your turn, Alex. What happened between you and Liam after little Connor arrived on the scene?"

Jenny didn't turn to look at Alex as she asked this, but Alex was impressed to realise that Jenny had bookmarked the point in her narrative where she had paused last time. It seemed a good sort of denouement for Alex to be producing at this point – the last quarter of the journey – when surely the driver must be tiring and should not be required to concentrate or respond to the events of the tale. It would be easy to interrupt the flow, too, when they reached the point where they had to start following Annie's email instructions to the letter, which was a matter of thirty miles or so now.

She glanced across at Jenny's calm expression, interpreted it as encouraging, and took up from where she had left off.

CHAPTER 8

The Last Stretch

"Oh yes – now, where was I? I think Liam was going off the rails a bit in Germany, wasn't he? We spent quite a lot of army life going backwards and forwards between Germany and England back then. There were to be a series of red flags for the marriage, which only a complete dunderhead would have ignored, but, of course, I sailed on regardless. One of the problems might have been that the nature of Army life at that time gave officers plenty of leeway to be heavy smokers and drinkers who might mess around with other women when doing a six month exercise here, or a year's posting there; it was a sort of Given, I suppose, in that disjointed way of working and living.

"It was the early Seventies, booze and fags were far cheaper than at home, and BBC and ITV television channels weren't yet available to British Army families in Europe. Perhaps that all contributed to the considerable number of parties where people got totally pissed and then created their own sexual crises, instead of being able to watch them on Soaps. No pot, though, Jenny, as far as I know. Being caught with it got you chucked out of the regiment straight away, which is funny really since most of the men – and some of their wives – were addling their brains with potentially more lethal amounts of alcohol.

"Anyway, Liam was an accomplished drinker. He was applauded for being able to drink up to sixteen double gin and tonics and still remain upright, if somewhat wobbly. I came to dread all such social functions over time, as his drinking habit became steadily more intense. I suppose he was unhappy, in retrospect, but in my 20's, I'm afraid that never really occurred to me. He was very proud of having won the Infantry Sword at Sandhurst, he was doing well in the regiment, he seemed popular enough, and it felt to me as if we were romantic with one another still. Well, I was certainly still in love with him; difficult to see exactly what was going wrong for him. Looking back on it, of course, our sex life could have been a lot more enterprising, but neither of us knew that at the time, as I've said.

"He no longer had to deny his Irish council house background, as he'd probably thought it necessary to do at Sandhurst, since he had joined an Irish regiment, and his upbringing now put him at grass roots camaraderie level with the men in his platoon. It seemed to me that he loved his easy familiarity of shared humour with them and vice versa. It gave him a big advantage over other junior officers who were English and not so au fait with the quirky foul mouthed innocence of Irish servicemen.

"He looked very good too in those days, despite all the booze and the fags, and maybe that was one of the problems. At the time of Beatle mania, he had very much the look of a young Paul McCartney; his soulful eyes, in particular. I think women gave him more than passing attention, and that was extremely heady stuff for his ego. He may, by now, have had his Irishness validated by the regiment, but it would be great to have his sexual attractiveness as a man, not a youth, validated too, and by 'worldly' women, not just by a fellow Enniskillen-er. He showed a particular vulnerability for a type of woman rarely seen in Fermanagh; tallish, slim but firmly built, with an auburn haired, freckled, wholesome look, whose way of speaking would be low-profile English, if you know what I mean – not posh.

"At the beginning of our married life, it was his drinking that worried me most but, to be fair, he wasn't particularly unpleasant when drunk in those first years, other than the odd burst of paranoid jealousy if we were having drinks in mixed company, and he thought someone was eyeing me up. (They never were, Jenny – I was at best mildly pretty, in an anxious sort of way.) He would normally be intent on having a good booze up with a mate or two, and I think that returning paralytic in the wee small hours was maybe part of the male bonding ritual. It worried me most because of a possible accident or fight or something; I didn't see it as a potential threat to our relationship at first.

"But things got worse once he was unhappy with a posting. He became adjutant to a colonel who had selected him for the job, but seemed, soon afterwards, to regret the choice, and they rapidly began to get on one another's nerves. This was pretty catastrophic because you've really got to get on with your boss, to some degree, if you are what amounts to his management interpreter and gofer. I think probably they were both from the same Ulster socially ambitious stock, and both could sense this about the other and despise it. Anyway, Liam was pretty much up against it during those two years in Germany, and developed a persecution mania in that work situation which wasn't entirely unjustified. As his drinking increased, I think the old demons must have begun to gnaw at him. Perhaps Colonel Swerve's distain for him triggered off memories of his own father's jealous contempt – I dunno. It wasn't that he had to bear it alone because his friends recognised what was happening and tried to support him, and I, of course, took every knock he endured to my heart, for his sake and my own.

"Well, he was rescued from that situation when a charismatic Irish general turned up and chose him for an upcoming posting as his personal assistant – his ADC – and swept us off to Lancashire for two years.

General Cathcart was a fine man and a much beloved soldier, greatly admired by one and all. I think one of the reasons he might have alighted on Liam as a possible choice was because the two men had a similar look to them – Irish charismatic charm! – and they were also about the same build. No average height General wants a beanpole of an ADC towering behind him! Anyway, the whole situation turned out exactly the opposite from Liam's previous experience as adjutant to the dreaded 'Swerve'. This time, the two of them, general and lieutenant, hit it off brilliantly and soon became devoted to one another. We were away from the regiment and stationed in a pretty quiet place which probably helped to foster a real friendship between the Cathcarts and us, despite the age and status difference.

"The general's wife, Penelope, was a reserved woman, brought up in Scotland, I think, with a real talent for decorative sewing, china restoration and delicate handicrafts of any sort, while I was a would-be maker of sellable trinkets. She had this motto, I remember, which seemed to apply to everything she did, whether as a mother, a general's wife, a dinner party hostess or an embroiderer – 'What I do, I do well.' This rather overwhelmed me at first, but one day we were talking about it, and I remarked to her that I thought my mum's rather more pragmatic motto, which I had adopted to some extent, was, 'What I do, I do quickly.' I remember that she threw back her head and laughed in a way that enchanted me, and we became friends from that day.

"That was a golden period for us, culminating in the month when Connor was born – the general became his godfather, naturally! – and when Liam's serving life was full of great stories, good boozing and a sense of being a surrogate son to the Cathcarts in some ways, along with their own beloved sons and daughter. You would have thought it would serve to wipe out the harm of the previous posting but, in retrospect, I see that it only arrested that deterioration for a while. Once the posting was at an end and we moved back to Germany, things should have been okay since there was a different commanding officer, and there were both old friends and new among the regiment; a much more benign regime all round.

"But I suppose Liam didn't feel specially selected any more. He was by now just a typical young captain within the regiment. I can't remember what role he had then, but it didn't seem to him to recognise his outstanding qualities as a young officer. He had won the Infantry Sword, after all, and, in his mind, he was thus obviously the best infantry man of his generation and should surely be acknowledged as top notch by his own regiment. Maybe it's like people who get four 'A's at 'A' level; once they get to university, that achievement doesn't get weighed against ordinary students like me with two 'B's or less, and the playing field becomes level again. I can see it must feel unfair to people who star at one stage, and Liam's starring at Sandhurst was a particularly bright event, given he was a rank outsider.

"So when he tried for the staff college exams once he was back in Germany again, he expected to pass first time, even though that was a rare achievement, unless you were an extremely high flyer indeed. If you did pass, it meant you would eventually be stationed in Camberley for two years and do more study, and then you could embark on the process of climbing up the army hierarchy beyond the rank of major towards becoming a field marshal and all that. You got three attempts at the staff college exams as a captain or a major, and the first failure shouldn't have stung Liam at the young age he was then, but it did. I think he couldn't bear to be 'normal'; it was absolutely normal to fail at your first attempt. So the drinking got worse, and, somehow, more aimed at escape than at drawing closer to his mates. I suppose he was becoming embittered somehow, as if he hadn't been given what was owing to him.

"I don't think he felt that bitterness about me and Connor – or if he did, it didn't really show up. Maybe he did feel it about me, comparing me with other sexier wives who were much more polished and accomplished, but he always retained some unfathomable sense of importance about my degree, regarding me as an intellectual because of it, and imagining I was thus, somehow, in that one area, a cut above some of the other wives. I wasn't very domesticated and my dinner parties usually served people a thinly disguised variation on mince and peas, but I wasn't actually a shame up for him; I could act the army wife role to a passable level, and Connor was, after all, the first born son and rather cute, if not always immaculately turned out.

"Liam was very sweet with him, though not particularly hands on about the daily maintenance. As Connor grew out of the baby phase, though, they became much closer. Liam was very good at inspiring Connor to try out new experiences, making an exciting adventure out of any new skill like riding a trike or swimming. So their bond began to strengthen, and even to withstand the many weeks separation here and there on army exercises; five months for one stint.

"Anyway, we were posted away again, this time for Liam to do some year-long course about weaponry in Dorset. He seemed pleased enough about it. As I've said, he had had a wobble or two, in terms of developing romantic yearnings towards one or two other women, which alarmed me a lot, but these seemed to pass over in a matter of months. There was quite a serious shake up with a neighbour's wife before we left Germany which had rocked the marriage badly, but we recovered from that, and he seemed more settled back in England among assorted men from a variety of service backgrounds and nationalities. Lots of us had young kids and, as a couple, we seemed at an advantage really, feeling at home in that part of England.

"But a strange thing happened. Half way through the course, Liam decided to apply for a two year posting as ADC within a small team of British officers advising the Nigerian Army; it would mean living in Kaduna, Northern Nigeria. I was doubtful about it, but I could see that things seemed to go wrong whenever Liam was back with his regiment, and I suppose I reckoned it might turn out differently in this set up out in Africa. Connor was still under four, I think, so it wouldn't disrupt his schooling at all, and we both knew nothing about Africa and thought it would be a great adventure. Am I boring you silly with all this, Jenny?"

"Not at all – I'm gripped!" replied Jenny brightly, smoothing her hair back from over her left ear.

"Well, the strange thing was that my brother James and his new-agey wife, Frances, were living not that far away in Wiltshire, at the time. And Frances was deeply into healing, and came over to stay with me to visit a psychic who was operating in some place like Bournemouth. We went off together and I had an appointment with this woman too, just to keep Fran company. I remember absolutely nothing about the consultation except that the woman suddenly looked very alarmed and said to me, 'Tell your husband he must not take up a job which involves crossing continents and living in a totally different climate. It will be disastrous if he does. Warn him not to take up any such opportunity.' She seemed really rather distressed.

"I remember I went back home to tell Liam, and to his credit, he was alarmed, too. We even talked about whether he could withdraw the application. However, it wasn't long afterwards that he heard he was to be offered the posting, and I suppose we both put the psychic's words to the back of our minds. He was doing well on the Bovington course, we had good friends there,

Connor was a cheerful little boy, we were even thinking of a second child...... I suppose I had kidded myself that Liam had been gradually maturing as a married man over his 20's, and was now moving into a more committed phase of family life, having belatedly sewn a few wild oats.

"I had stupidly believed his story of not actually having had sex with the neighbour's wife in Germany, auburn haired and charmingly English, of course. She had been replayed to me as simply a crush, not to be brought up again. Much later, just as he was leaving me, Liam confessed that he had lied about this and that she had, he claimed, persuaded him into passionate sex on a number of occasions. He only volunteered the truth about all this because, faced with the break-up of the family, I had finally questioned him directly as to when his infidelities had first started in the marriage. By then he had nothing to lose by being honest about his various dalliances, and he probably told me something pretty close to the truth. But I'm jumping about in the story — sorry!

"So off we went to Nigeria. Liam hated it within six weeks of arrival. He loathed his commanding officer, and resented the fact that he was little more than a lackey to him and to the entire team of high powered colonels who were serving alongside him. They all lived in rather splendid accommodation in a private enclave near the military HQ and we had a much smaller bungalow in the grounds of the C.O.'s spacious residence. To be honest, I came to like life there more and more as time went by. We all suffered from the frequent lengthy power cuts, whether we lived in mansions or bungalows. Electricity or the lack of it was no respecter of income, unless you were one of the few people who owned a generator. So domestic arrangements were unpredictable, and I rather enjoyed the uncertainty and randomness about life there, which all of us shared.

"The heat could be searing and the humidity frightful, but there was many a jovial party in the gardens, and I liked the other wives and their kids, and felt at home enough among them. We were all provided with servants at minimal cost, and having a steward and a gardener meant that life was luxurious in many ways. Our steward, Miriam, adored Connor and he, her. Our gardener, Abdu, was a great character, not too keen on gardening but excellent value in entertainment and local knowledge. Their presence gave me freedom to take up things I wanted to do in the area occasionally, as Connor seemed just as happy in their company as in mine, if it was necessary to leave him behind for a couple of hours.

"I think what I liked best was the multi-national, ex pat community and the way we army folk could swiftly be integrated into their various circles. It was quite different from how army couples might feel in Britain, where cultivating 'civilian friends' was an acquired art. I soon became a member of the International Women's Club, a group of earnest women who provided linen for outlying clinics or raised money for play parks in orphanages. I also taught every morning at a local Nursery school and came to love it. Connor came along too, when he felt like it, and he seemed at home in my class. He was made very welcome by staff and pupils alike, even though he was the only white child there. I don't think I ever got to know any Nigerians as close friends, I'm afraid, apart from Miriam and Abdu, but I came to know various professional people outside our little army life who might be navigating successfully between Kaduna's tribal communities and the new economic entrepreneurs who were cashing in on oil.

"This kind of freedom of movement into the community, even if I was experiencing it sort of by proxy, wasn't so available to our husbands, and I think Liam's role provided the least possible job satisfaction because he wasn't even involved in the training of Nigerian officers and soldiers – just facilitating the domestic arrangements of those British officers who were. He was endlessly tied up in trying to arrange travel details for various officers' kids travelling between their boarding schools in U.K. and Nigeria.

"Back then, Nigerian bureaucracy was, at best, intricate and complex and, at worst, downright obstructionist or even corrupt. Liam came to scorn everything about life there, however exciting it had first seemed to us as newcomers. His hatred of it all extended beyond the lepers who ambushed him outside the bank and the officials who simultaneously condemned and courted bribery to include, eventually, the story book African mud hut villages in the bush or the magnificent colours adorning the vibrant market place crowd. It was all toxic to him in the end.

"We decided that I would plead particular medical need to return to Britain for the birth of our second child. No such clinical need existed at all, but I had had an insignificant miscarriage in our first months out there, and we seized upon the excuse of the supposed trauma of this event to opt for seeing through the next pregnancy to its nine month conclusion back home.

"It seemed a clever wheeze for Liam to have the hope of a temporary escape from Nigeria, in the form of a week's compassionate leave in Northern Ireland, to be there at my side where our second baby was to be born. The only drawback was that it meant Connor and I would have to leave Liam in Kaduna some time before the due birth date as there were limits to how late on in a pregnancy I was allowed by the airline to fly. I was worried about how Liam would cope without us, as he seemed to be on the edge of some sort of breakdown. However, he assured me that the prospect of that week of compassionate leave away from Kaduna in May would be enough to keep him going through March and April and then, subsequently, until the whole wretched posting finished.

"It wasn't. Within a week of my departure for Northern Ireland, he was, I learnt later, deeply involved with Helen, wife of one of the colonels in the team, and the two of them deserted their spouses and children and their way of life within a very short period, sailing off into the sunset together. You can guess how Helen looked, dear Jenny! Her copper coloured hair and smiling, freckled face were not suited to the Nigerian climate, as she needed to protect herself from harsh sunlight but she was, nonetheless, the sort of woman who smelt of fresh air, stood tall, and glowed with outdoor health. She was eight years older than Liam, but you'd never have known it. I bet the romance set that little British community on fire with sensational gossip but I was long gone, and never around again, thank goodness, to experience it!

"Liam had to make a brief visit to Ireland in order to put stuff of his in storage and that sort of thing. He saw the boys at that time but it didn't seem possible for him to find any way of relating to me as a co parent or even as a long term friend. He was utterly fixated on his new relationship with Helen and behaved like a total stranger with me, as if he was encased in ice. It was during that time, as I've said, that I'd sneaked a look at one of his letters from Helen when he was on the phone, and realised from her passionate expressiveness about their sex life that I was completely outclassed and out of the running.

"As soon as I could, I got the boys away from my camping with Liam's parents and joined my own folks who happened to be living in New Orleans at the time. (My mum had influential relations there who had arranged a superb pastor job for Dad after his retirement from his headship; he was standing in for a minister who was on a four year international project.) All four parents were horrified, of course, at this disastrous turn of events, but Liam was out of touch and there was nothing much anyone could do. After three months in the States, I decided to return to Britain and start a new life for myself and the children, in London. I flew back to Heathrow from New Orleans on a night flight on 31st December, 1979. It seemed to me like a good omen to be flying into a new life and a new decade simultaneously, but, of course, a cheap stand by flight had been much more likely to be available on New Year's Eve than at other times, which is actually why I happened to be flying that night!

"I knew that Social Services would accommodate me in some sort of hostel as a single parent with two young children, and I guessed I could get a teaching job. I was very lucky that things worked out well for me. I had a dear friend from university days living in London with her husband, and they put me up initially, refusing to hear of me going into any sort of emergency accommodation. They went on to support me in every possible way, allowing me and the boys to stay on with them despite the very limited accommodation and the inconvenience for them, until I found my feet again. Against their wishes, I was just about able to contribute financially to staying there because my generous American relatives had given me tide-over money, which I could accept as a gift or eventually repay, as I chose.

"Within a year, I was settled in a little upstairs flat in Lewisham with the boys, thanks to my parents lending me the money to buy it. I had a good job teaching English in a local Comprehensive, which paid me enough to manage fine and to start monthly repayments to my parents, and to save towards repaying the American debt. Things were so much easier for me financially than they were for you! Gradually, I built up a small network of great people, through my friends in the English department, who were changing my world with me and for me. But I was heartbroken. It took me at least ten years to get over it. Certainly, I would sometimes have liked to stop living but there were the kids – you had to go on for them – you know how it was.

"I think Connor was even more devastated than I was. His primary teacher told me she had never seen a child sadder than him. Wee Paddy, of course, had scarcely encountered his father. So there would not, I hoped, be the same impact of loss once he was old enough to realise he had no resident dad. All I could do was try to guide Connor through the loss; recognise it, share it, but make the best of our new London life together. I tried never to cry in front of him. I didn't want a five year old thinking he had to be strong for me and his baby brother. Gradually, we began to love London. It was an exciting place to be in the early Eighties, and our little family began to find its secure place within the city.

"Liam and Helen eventually emerged from their halcyon bubble, and resurfaced in Yorkshire. They began to have both boys for extended visits each summer. Liam requested a speedy divorce – I suppose Helen did, too – and both rejected partners obliged. I think Liam and Helen genuinely sought to bring her teenage kids and his much younger ones back to a new sort of stability, despite their abrupt departure from the respective families. It certainly helped Connor to recover; I'm not sure what it did for Pad at such a young age, but Helen was a devoted stepmother both to him and to Connor, and the two boys themselves were always very close. I think Pad probably suffered from being the 'afterthought son', as far as Liam was concerned, and I am eternally grateful that Helen did her best to protect Paddy very lovingly when the light of Liam's attention shone particularly warmly on Connor during their annual visits

"I think Helen's own two teenagers were old enough to give their mum a pretty rough time when they were staying with her and their newly acquired stepfather, whom they both intensely resented from the start. I think the younger of the two, Katie, was more subtly subversive than her brother, but together they must gradually have formed an increasingly effective opposition to the whole relationship.

They were regularly present during those Yorkshire summers, in any case, and were endlessly warm and patient with their new young stepbrothers. Maybe Connor and Pad gradually began to gain by their immersion in two separate worlds – I hope so, anyway.

"Liam occasionally wrote me sharp letters about the inadequate discipline routines and general standards in the boys' London home life, but he did his best to support them financially on a regular basis, after he eventually found civilian employment. He seemed to hate me. Later, I began to understand that it was more that he hated the thought of me. His turn around and desertion had never really surprised me. At some level, I think I'd always known in my heart of hearts that he didn't love me. I didn't blame him or Helen for what had happened. I never asked, 'Why me?'

"Actually, I now felt at one with other people who had had something hard to deal with, whereas before, I had been all too guiltily aware of how easy my life had been for me. I had come to love my teaching job, and I much admired the tough London kids who shaped my strategies in the classroom by their good natured derision and wit. I liked being a civilian, I think! I used to smile at the Army Reject shop in fellow feeling, but I reckoned that somehow, maybe I'd been lucky to have been jettisoned out of that strange itinerant life. Now, perhaps, I would at last learn to be my Self, if I was at all capable of that.

"Looking back on it, I see that I fell far short of it. I got our lives back up together, found a career, stabilised things to some extent for the boys, gave them back as much of their father as he was offering them, discounted bitterness, and worked on my own happiness by meeting and attempting to connect with Dan. I never quite clicked on the Self bit though, because I don't think I ever really understood how much I had lost my identity within Liam's. If I'd known then what we know now!"

"Better late than never, though, isn't it?" mused Jenny, with a rueful nod.

"Yeah. I guess I'm just a slow learner!" With a brief wriggle of her shoulders, Alex shifted her back's position against the back of her seat and adjusted her propped up knees yet again. "We'll get there, won't we, Jenny? Just before the early onset Alzheimer's kicks in!"

"Not so early at our age, Alex!" came the swift reply and now it was Alex's turn to smile, with eyes glancing upward, mouth corners downward for a moment. Yet she knew for certain that neither of them would ever fear neurological decay either imminently or in the distant future. Those who fight as long as they had done to regain sanity would never knowingly lose it again, and if they must lose it unknowingly, how could that distress them? A sense of exuberance hit her suddenly.

"No more abandonment fears for us, remember; we're beyond all that. We're free to live our life *in* abandonment, and sanity just doesn't come into it!"

"Amen to that!" laughed Jenny, with a brief jubilant wiggle of the steering wheel.

CHAPTER 9

Arrival

The light on the surrounding hillsides was laced with a gentle gold as they began negotiating the series of winding, narrow lanes which were taking them towards Annie's 'Daydreams'. Her directions were easy to follow, and Jenny had some residual memory of the terrain she had covered a year ago when approaching the Bed and Breakfast accommodation for the first time.

This winning combination meant that they were driving up to the yellow gate soon after six o'clock, without having lost their way at any point. Both women had been fully engaged in the business of route negotiation for at least forty minutes, and found themselves somewhat dazed to have actually reached their goal. They needed to make the switch to being outside the motionless car, on firm ground, and about to launch into an unfamiliar sort of social interaction.

"We'll leave the bags in the back, shall we?" Jenny glanced over to Alex, assuming she would concur with this move towards an unencumbered initial encounter. Alex nodded, and they stood beside the car for a moment, reluctant to make the first move towards the front door.

"Very peaceful, isn't it?" Jenny commented, as both women looked back along the lane that ran up to and beyond the house. The hedgerow opposite bordered a hilly field, and there were two higher points of land to their right, beyond the crossroads where they had turned to mount the slope towards Annie's place. Sheep grazed beyond five bar gates, and the grass, shrubbery and trees were lush with every shade of green. Birds were singing and from somewhere distant came the intermittent barking of a dog, but there was no sound of traffic.

"And it's not even raining!"

Alex had not often seen rural Wales in these pleasant conditions and had to admit to herself that she was surprised by its jaunty, sunlit hills. It had the look of a child's colouring book, illustrating The Countryside; the sort of printed drawing which, as a small child, she would once have started to colour in, using a tiny bordering line of yellow along the horizon edges.

"We'll probably have time for an evening stroll once we've got ourselves sorted out," remarked Jenny, more to herself than to Alex. "Stretch the old legs a bit! You realise we've covered almost three hundred miles today? It's good to be out of the car, isn't it?" As she was speaking, Jenny laid a hand on the bonnet of her Nissan Micra, almost as if she was trying to counterbalance any negative effect of her comment. The car appeared to be making a quiet clicking noise from underneath somewhere, in acknowledgement. There was a pause.

"Well, I expect we'd better knock."

Jenny moved somewhat reluctantly towards the beautifully manicured front of the house.

Alex stepped behind her and waited on the gravel path as Jenny reached the three stone steps up to the front door, painted a shiny golden yellow.

"Do you think we should close that?" Alex asked, nodding back towards the entrance gate which had allowed them open access to drive into the parking area.

"Well, it was open when we arrived. There may be other people staying too. I think we'd better just leave it as it is."

Alex nodded. There was another pause. Jenny remained at the base of the first step.

Both women glanced up in surprise as the heavy door suddenly opened and a pleased voice announced, "Oh, here you are! Well done! You found me!"

The speaker came down the steps to greet Jenny with a hug. Jenny motioned Alex forward to be introduced to Annie, and all three women stood smiling at one another in the space between the garage wall and the front steps.

"Let's bring in your things to the porch for now, shall we?" suggested their hostess, and they complied efficiently, collecting their overnight bags from the boot of the car. Once inside the spacious porch, they deposited the bags in the corner indicated and stepped through into the large living room. A quick glance round confirmed Alex's expectation of décor perfection, down to the last detail. However, there was a note of contrast in the dog bed lodged close to the giant sofa, where a sickly looking terrier was lying, attempting to yelp in a strangled sort of way. A bowl of water was positioned near its mouth, on top of old newspaper, and there was a heavy scent of Roses room spray.

"This is Carla. I hope you don't mind her being here, but she is very poorly and I need to keep an eye on her." Annie's brow was etched with anxiety, and both visitors attempted to assume the same sort of facial expression.

"Oh dear! What's the matter with her?" asked Jenny, with polite concern.

"Well, it's mainly old age, I'm afraid. She had a growth there between her front legs and that was operated on last year and removed. It wasn't actually cancerous but the vet warned me back then that he would have to put her on long term medication and that I must...."

Alex tuned out from the account of Carla's health problems and took in more of her surroundings. There were huge patio doors leading out into a beautifully arranged garden, the white conservatory peeping out to the left, the borders a riot of flowers and blended shrubbery. Two white wooden benches were positioned on the edge of the lawn, and a water feature constructed from small, tumbling rocks glistened between them. It all had the air of a retreat; a haven crafted for the owner and her guests to appreciate quiet beauty and to be healed by the sanctuary it provided.

Alex felt vaguely uncomfortable and turned away from the window to look at the four large, dark oil paintings on the wall opposite the patio doors. The paintings were of pink, yellow and red roses, somewhat faded and overblown, with the odd petal poised to fall. They were impressive works of art which lived up to their tastefully ornate frames. Their formal elegance provided an air of gravitas to what was otherwise a living space frothing with pastels, frills, tassels and pleats. It crossed Alex's mind that the general look of the room was much more expensive than one might expect for a small Welsh guest house, and she had to remind herself that Annie's charges were actually perfectly reasonable.

She tuned back into the conversation going on near the ailing Carla, which had now moved on to the health of Annie's two cats. Alex had never owned an animal and felt equally unable to participate in this new aspect of the topic, but as Jenny had owned a beloved tabby herself, there was now a livelier two way communication going on about the relationship between Agas and cats; a very positive one, apparently. The mention of the Aga seemed to lead naturally to the welcome offer of a cup of tea at the kitchen table.

Half an hour later, after tea and coffee had been sipped from bone china mugs, home-made cake had been consumed, and a tour of the garden and the recently completed conservatory had been accomplished, Jenny and Alex were mounting the staircase to their bedroom. They paused in the landing alcove to marvel, yet again, at Annie's skills in soft furnishings. They assured their hostess that they needed no help with their overnight bags, and were soon at the top of the stairs, just outside their allocated bedroom.

As Annie turned to leave her guests, both women thanked her simultaneously and Alex added,

"It's all so luxurious! It's more like a five star hotel than a Bed and Breakfast!"

This remark seemed to hit a nerve, as Annie immediately stopped in her tracks.

"Well, I do think it's crazy to rate this accommodation as two star, but that's all I can ever achieve here because neither guest bedroom is en suite. You have your guest bathroom just opposite and a separate loo but, of course, if the other bedroom was booked – which it isn't – you'd have to share those facilities. I could pave the walls and ceiling with solid gold tiles and I'd still only ever gain two stars because of that. It seems absolutely daft to me."

Both women nodded sympathetically.

"And I am not willing to destroy the character of an eighteenth century farmhouse by putting in a ridiculous amount of additional plumbing, just to tick the boxes of the Tourist Provision Inspection Gestapo. I love this place too much to submit to those bureaucratic philistines who would rather butcher a much treasured space, maintained lovingly over centuries, than ask a tourist to step across a hallway for a wee wee. The sort of people who come to stay here always seem to share my values rather than theirs, and surely those are the sort of tourists this country needs."

Jenny and Alex again indicated their support for this group of adaptable urinators. There was a moment's silence.

"So – um – are we able to have supper with you tonight? queried Jenny tentatively. "It doesn't matter at all if it doesn't suit. It's just we really would appreciate a chance at some point to talk with you about this little project of ours. I know you said we could eat in the pub in the next village, but would you be able to join us?"

"Oh yes! My friend Bianca wants to come as well. I mentioned that, didn't I, in my email? The only thing is, we must get there by eight as they stop serving by half past. It's just basic food of course, nothing special, but it's all there is around here. I'm afraid we aren't spoilt for choice in this area, as far as sophisticated dining is concerned. I'm happy to drive, and we can pick up Bianca on our way. We were both very intrigued by what you wrote, Jenny. I gather you are trying to do some research into the nature of dangerous relationships, or something like that? Bianca is a writer, you know. She might well be able to offer some very useful support and guidance."

"Gosh! A published writer, you mean?" asked Alex.

"Yes, and a very successful one. She has written two books about collies as working dogs which were very popular reading in Wales. I think she took up that subject after she had at least three cookery books published, one after the other; the third of them made quite a lot of money for her. You'll be able to ask her about how she got into it all. Are you hoping to get something published? Is it Non Fiction? Because I think Bianca would have quite a bit to offer by way of advice, if you'd like that."

"Well, we don't quite know where we going with the stuff we've gathered so far. It's just a few notes, really." Alex was keen to distance herself rapidly from literary professionalism. "Um, we're really only at the research stage right now, and needing your help about – er – well, just about actual experience."

"Well, we are looking forward to hearing about it all."

Annie seemed to have regained her composure, and she was turning once again towards the stairs as she continued, "I'll leave you in peace for now, and perhaps we could set off from here at about quarter to eight? I did take the precaution of booking a table for the four of us. If you wanted an evening stroll before that, you could just wander out the front and leave the door open. There's no need for a key or anything. Poor old Carla's not going anywhere, in her present state. I don't think you'll have time to get lost, but if you do, remember that we're up the hill past the old Primary school building at the crossroads."

"Yes, I think we will have a little dander," said Jenny, shrugging her shoulders up and down, while tipping back her neck. "The driving wasn't bad at all, and we had no traffic hold ups, but all the same, it is a relief to be stretching our limbs and looking forward to a breath of fresh air. Thank you very much for booking a table; that's great. And pub grub is just the job! We weren't holding out for haute cuisine!"

"Well, it's not even pub grub as you'd probably think of it in the South; more like fry ups or fiery curries. But I don't do an evening meal here for guests, as a rule, because I used to get exhausted with that if I was doing full English breakfasts in the morning as well. Would you be wanting those, incidentally?"

"Not at all!" declared Alex quickly, while Jenny shook her head firmly to endorse the words.

Annie nodded, and proceeded to list the breakfast alternatives she could provide at any time they wanted in the morning, up until ten o'clock. Smiling at the enthusiastic gratitude of her two guests, she stepped away with a final nod. After a few moments, Jenny stepped forward and closed the door quietly from the inside.

"Wow!" intoned Alex as she dived head first onto the bed beside the window, her face immediately buried within two king sized pillows. Jenny repositioned her bag on the bed she had claimed, the same one she had slept in the previous year, and sat down heavily, with a sigh of relief.

"Is it okay, Alex?" she asked after a moment, as there was no sign of resurfacing from the pillows opposite. Alex shifted position, emerged and rolled over onto her back.

"It's incredible!" Alex exclaimed, giggling a little. "It's sort of New Age Chic. I've never seen those two styles combined in quite this way. And Annie's pretty unexpected, too; certainly not a hint of a victim about her."

"You had imagined a more downtrodden type, had you?" enquired Jenny, with interest.

"Well, you'd told me she was an air hostess in her 20's. That's how she got involved with her Narcissist, isn't it? He was a pilot? It surprises me that you can still sense such glamour about her and that she is still lovely to look at, so many years later: perfect features, superb make up and meticulous attention to detail, right down to her delicately manicured, crescent shaped fingernails. You know what I mean? That immaculate cream silk blouse and perfectly tailored skirt! She's everything I could never be."

"Yes, she looks exceedingly good. And she can't be all that much younger than us! It's such an advantage being tall and having excellent deportment. But I think she does look her age somehow because of the down turn of her mouth; she doesn't look a happy lit'l ol' bunny, does she?"

"No, she doesn't," agreed Alex. "But those deep green eyes of hers are amazing. And did you notice her eyelashes, Jenny? D'you think they're false? They go on for ever. If they are false, I can't believe she bought ones as good as that in darkest Wales. But I have a horrible feeling they are real. She must have been devastatingly beautiful when she was younger."

"You probably had to be that good looking, to be an air hostess back then. I think it was seen as a very glamorous profession initially; quite a contrast to the low cost flight attendant sort of idea nowadays. I suppose it was because flying used to be a much more elitist form of travel than it is today, when we're all peppering the skies with our carbon foot prints, and warming up the ice caps. Anyway, Alex, how about a stroll? We haven't much more than half an hour before we set off for a culinary extravaganza at the pub. Are you up for a wander or would you prefer to stay in here for a while?"

"Nope – I'm raring to go," said Alex, levering herself off the bed. And shortly afterwards, both women were making their way out of the open front door and into the lane, facing the evening sun.

Alex was surprised to find herself grateful for the sunset walk they had taken once she and Jenny later found themselves at the entrance of a green and grey public house beside a village garage. Somehow, the street had an oppressive effect on her, even though the straggle of dreary buildings on either side of it was broken up, and of no great length. Things felt little better as they stepped inside. Jenny was talking to Bianca, and Annie had gone up to the bar to establish where their booked table was to be found. Alex gazed around her, and was reminded, suddenly and unaccountably, of unhappy days in her Dublin boarding school.

Annie soon returned to usher her three companions to a small dark round table in the eating area of the lounge. There were no other diners on the four other tables but there were two small groups of drinkers positioned much nearer the bar, some of whom seemed to have remnants of nuts and crisps in front of them. One or two people from these circles glanced over at the four quiet women as they took up their position at the furthest corner of the room. It would, however, have taken a very penetrating stare to make out the facial expressions of any of the women taking their seats because the eating area was dimly lit, as if to discourage patrons from requesting the evening menu.

Alex was grateful for the inadequate light. She guessed it would probably fall to her to introduce the topic uniting them round the table, and she felt suddenly uncomfortable, uncertain of what words to use. She knew Jenny wanted her to be the one to explain exactly why they had come. It was difficult to guess how a more detailed description of their mission might be received by their two fellow diners.

She had noticed that Annie seemed pleased to have been the chauffeur and was content to relax, now that the reserved table had been acquired and some service was likely to be provided. She had seemed cheered even before that, from the point when Bianca had been waiting outside her house to be picked up, and had greeted her friend affectionately as she climbed into the front seat. But as Annie had waved a hand backwards to introduce Alex and Jenny to her, Bianca had turned round to smile at them, two strangers, with exactly the same warmth of easy familiarity as she had used to salute her close friend. She was a broad shouldered woman with carefully cut, mid length grey hair and a strong, intelligent face. Looking across to her now, Alex wondered whether there was actually no need for any nervousness. Bianca seemed the sort of person whose presence was essentially reassuring.

A teenage girl in a copious white blouse came to take their order, apologising for various items listed on the menu but now unavailable. Alex had already established that she and Jenny would pay for the meal which meant that, as well as taking the orders, the waitress was asked to bring a bottle of white wine, a contribution from the other pair of women. Two fish and chips, a tuna salad and a burger bap with French fries were ordered from the menu. The waitress had only just turned towards the kitchen when Bianca smiled across at Alex and raised her eyebrows, one hand stretched out.

"Annie and I are so intrigued to know more about what you are doing," she said, glancing over towards her friend as she spoke. "Please go ahead when you're ready to begin."

Alex giggled momentarily, shooting a wry smile in Jenny's direction. "Oh dear! I'm not sure *how* to begin! It's very good of you both to be prepared to go along with us, and give us your time." She glanced across at Jenny and then cleared her throat slightly before speaking again. "Well, I suppose the story starts with the fact that Jenny and I taught at the same Southampton Girls' Inner City Comprehensive for more than a decade, since around 1985, I think, wasn't it? We weren't close friends – not in the same department – but we knew enough about each other to know we had both been abruptly left, as young wives, with two small children.

"I had eventually remarried, moving from London to Hampshire, and had got a chance for a new family life, with a trio of kids, because my two boys acquired a beloved sister in my husband Dan's little daughter, Bella. As for Jenny; what would you say about yourself after Joe, Jenny?"

"Well, I was lucky because the close friends I had living nearby after my husband left were so encouraging that I got the confidence to have a second crack at art college, as a mature student on a government grant. I went on to do teacher training afterwards, and eventually I was able to start a new career as an Art teacher, and to rebuild my life on much better foundations."

Jenny looked a little uncomfortable and her tone was crisp as she filled in this information. Alex gathered that she did not particularly want to be brought into the story directly at this point. She took up the narrative again herself.

"So – um – there we were, both of us, with our teaching jobs and our apparently settled lives. But somehow, I eventually got myself into a state of clinical depression and had to be medically evacuated out of the school, after fifteen years there. I was so ashamed of myself, but there was nothing I could do really but accept my colossal disgrace, and the generous early retirement pay out, and move on to another line of work. My husband, Dan, was great and so were all my family and friends and eventually, within a year, I got a voluntary job helping out on an Arts project.

"The professor in charge was a handsome, very charming, somewhat self-obsessed sort of man and I thought I'd got the measure of him, though I was rather enchanted by our sparkling repartee; he was a brilliant mimic, and I have never laughed so much as I did in the first months of working for him. But within a year or two, somehow my whole being had got enmeshed in him. Eventually, he left the job rather suddenly, under a bit of a cloud. I think it was something to do with seriously inappropriate internet use, or breaching copyright – all pretty dodgy but I never found out exactly what.

"It was all kept very hush-hush because of the risk of adverse publicity for the whole project which depended largely on generous U.S. funding. I was mates with the secretary to the site manager, and she knew all about the bills for computer network maintenance – I certainly remember some whispers about importing 'filth' and a resulting virus but at that time, I had no idea what those words indicated technically. Marcus himself said the trustees had decided to get rid of him because he was too much sought after personally on his American fund raising lectures, and this had ruffled feathers among the major financiers of the project.

"Anyway, he and I stayed in close touch for a further year which wasn't that difficult because we lived within ten miles of one another, and he was now working from his home on his next book, and I carried on doing research for him. I had got pretty used to trawling through all sorts of Victorian Literature by that time. But then he abruptly decided to cut off contact with me. We were both married, and he must have concluded it was best to end the friendship there and then. And that was that. I then found myself thrown back in a strange new version of the original depression. I stayed on working for the Arts project, now as a low paid member of staff, since my role had been switched to a sort of Education Officer there.

"Well, at this stage, Jenny and I were just beginning to meet about a joint educational venture we were planning, using her Special Needs Year eleven students to do sculptures based round the idea of hidden treasures. (The school Jenny had moved to after she had left our Girls' school was quite near Uplands House, where I was working.) You remember that hidden hoard of Bailey's poems and letters that turned up a few years back? There was a lot of publicity about it back then. That was at Uplands.

"Back in Victorian times, there had been a secret romance between the owners' young daughter, Rose, and James Bailey. All this came to light when the house was being renovated. Soon afterwards, considerable funding became available from the States, through the U.S. Bailey Society, to buy the house from the hotel developers who had acquired it, and turn it instead into a research centre based round the 'Literature of Romance'. It had been Marcus's role, as director, to match the U.S. funding in Britain and Europe, and to promote the centre as a unique research facility and conference base.

"Anyway, I remember this so well! Jenny and I were sitting in a pub one lunch time, planning out how we'd handle the project with her school kids, using the back of a beer mat for notes. Once we'd finished, we began to talk about other things, and I asked her how her heart was. We'd sort of lost touch a bit when she'd gone off to Ireland for a while, and of course, I'd subsequently gone off the rails mentally! I knew that this guy, Ricky, had been living with her, apparently blissfully, for quite a few years, but that the relationship had broken up some time previously, leaving Jenny shocked and uncomprehending. I suppose it was intrusive of me to ask, but once you've gone crazy yourself and lost your whole job infrastructure, you tend not to be so cautious any more, if you know what I mean....."

"I didn't find it intrusive," commented Jenny quickly. "It was just a hard question to answer. Everyone I knew, family and friends, had been shocked and then very sympathetic when I'd finally discovered that Ricky had a Spanish lover on the go, and I realised that I had, latterly at least, just been a staging post for his moving on to her. But a year further on, they were presuming I'd got over it; good riddance, sort of. It was a bit startling to have someone actually ask me about my traumatised heart."

She lowered her head again. Alex was observing the other pair of women as Jenny spoke, and noticed that they were both leaning forward slightly, clearly attentive. Indeed, all four women were surprised by the reappearance of the waitress at this point, with wine glasses, the white wine, and sets of cutlery wrapped in dark green paper napkins. There was a pause as the bottle was opened, glasses and wine distributed, and cutlery passed round.

"Carry on, please," said Bianca, nodding at Alex, who was a little hesitant about continuing her narrative. She nodded in response, thankful for Bianca's encouragement.

"Well, what Jenny answered was something like – er – she was just a hologram of herself. Wasn't that it, Jenny? And that response sort of rang a bell with me. Because, by now, I was in my last year at the Arts project job, and I was also training to be a counsellor. I had, some months before, come across a chapter – compulsory homework reading! – about the effect of either too much or too little attention on a very young child. There had been a list of possible types of damage which might occur as a result, and one of the words which cropped up was 'narcissistic'.

"I remember reading it and being surprised that such a trendy word, apparently used in common parlance to describe someone who was stuck up about his or her appearance, should be employed in this serious psychology article. So, out of idle curiosity, I googled the word and, among all the thousands of related hits that came up, there was this phrase, here and there, 'Narcissistic Personality Disorder'. I'd never heard of it, and I was intrigued enough to follow through the links. I eventually fell upon a set of nine descriptors defining the disorder itself.

"As I began to read through them, I suddenly felt myself transfixed by the list on the screen because, as I read down, almost every single one of those nine criteria was fitting my professor Marcus to a tee. The matching totally dumbfounded me! I realised that by sheer chance, I had tumbled upon an almost perfect description of Marcus's internal state of being. It hit me, then and there, that I had allowed myself to fall into the mind set of disorder alongside him and *that* was why I was depressed again. I realised that I had foolishly risked the loss of my marriage and my whole stable family life in order to step aboard the roller coaster of another person's idealising fantasies.

"Anyway...." Alex tried to lighten her tone. "Er, because Jenny had used that hologram phrase, it sounded to me as if she might actually be in the same sort of mental state that I was. The two men were entirely different in looks, demeanour and modus operandi and at first, I simply couldn't imagine that her tall, charismatic Irishman with his exuberant jokes and his hearty joie de vivre, so different in personality from my compact, perfectionist professor, would possibly similarly qualify as someone far along the Narcissistic spectrum, but that didn't seem to be the point.

"It sounded as if we both had been similarly affected by our relationships with these two men. It suddenly struck me to wonder whether we were both somehow caught in the slipstream of relationship dysfunction, and couldn't really recover because we hadn't accurately identified what was wrong with us."

She glanced at her listeners and was relieved to see that Annie was nodding in affirmation, glass to her lips.

"So really, that's the essence of our story, such as it is. Over the many months that followed, we began to piece things together about the young men we had married and the second pair of men we had fallen for in our 40's or 50's. And I think we began to make some sense of it, which had been particularly challenging for me since I, after all, was long married, by now, to a good man who loved me and had done everything he could to support me through the school disaster thing. How could I have betrayed such a man for someone who was fundamentally just a player?

"I remember that when I first read that list of nine traits in one of the Narcissistic Personality Disorder sites, I had run straight into the other room and told my husband about it, in a state of high excitement. Dan wasn't that interested, naturally, but I suppose I felt sort of vindicated because I had all along tried to describe my relationship with Marcus as honestly as I could to him. I used to say to Dan, 'I don't understand what is going on between me and Marcus – he just somehow fills me with a sort of wild childlike joy, sometimes; as if we were jamming with magical harmonies. But I'd never want to live with him; he's somehow from another world. My love for him is nothing like my love for you. I could never, ever imagine my life without you in it.'

"Anyway, Dan was somewhat perplexed while it was going on, my stuff with Marcus, but he did not appear to be unduly worried. I think he thought it was intellectual masturbation of some kind, two English Literature wankers, with a bit of hero worship thrown in. My husband is a very reserved man, you see, extremely self sufficient emotionally, and without any obvious need for intimacy of any sort. He is also pretty distrustful of verbal eloquence!

"Actually, his natural reticence, being the shy middle brother among two male siblings, was greatly augmented by too many rather savage years at boarding school; he learnt to be pretty mistrustful of confiding feelings in anyone, as a result. He may not have revealed any heartfelt response to my encounters with Marcus, but I certainly knew that he thought Marcus was an odious little man. I remember he'd say, 'No wonder you two enjoy each other's company so much; you both adore Professor Marcus!'

"There was one time when I came back from a picnic with Marcus, and told Dan about it, as usual; this time, I explained about where we'd found a lovely spot in the sun. I remember adding with some pride, pointing to my suntanned shoulders and arms,

'And Marcus says I'm amazingly long-limbed.' Dan, who's tall and skinny, snorted in derision and remarked, 'Everyone's long-limbed to a munchkin!'"

Alex paused as the others chuckled along with her.

"But occasionally, Dan also used to warn me of danger. I remember once he said to me, 'If you ever go off with Marcus, his wife will recover, I will be fine, Marcus will sail through, whatever happens, but *you* will destroy yourself.' He could see it all so clearly – amazing, isn't it?"

Alex was at her most anxious at this point of the narrative, aware that sexual infidelity, though unstated, might well be assumed and condemned by her listeners. If so, they displayed no evidence of it. The arrival of their ordered meals provided another break in the story. Alex eventually took up the thread again.

"I've always been a bit obsessive, and gradually, I began reading everything I could get my hands on about Personality Disorder. Well, actually, it wasn't about all sorts of personality dysfunction; I was only interested in researching the ones which had the biggest impact on personal relationships. I'm afraid I used to do so initially as a sort of sublimation because I felt so bereft without Marcus in my life any more. I somehow got close to him again through all the reading which so often described the sort of things he said and did, though only indirectly, of course.

"Often, I could make very little sense of it. I had no training in Psychology, it was complex reading with lots of technical terms, and I couldn't find anyone else who knew much about it to help me. So poor Jenny bore the brunt of my research and very gradually, we began to match up bits of what I was finding out – if I understood it – with things we had both actually experienced in our two key damaging relationships with two men each. And after a very long time of doing this, I suppose… well, what could we say, Jenny?"

"Well, maybe we began to notice that we were getting a fraction saner!"

"Only a fraction, though." They both smiled at this proviso. Jenny suddenly took up the tale.

"And then it all sort of began to expand a bit, and we imagined we could spot when other people we met were in the sustained shocked state that we had been in, and hadn't recognised it, any more than we had. And we sort of realised that these shocked people could be sons or daughters or friends or husbands or wives or fathers or mothers or employees or absolutely anyone who had been born or drawn into a relationship which they hadn't cottoned on to being dysfunctional."

"Oh, I see!" exclaimed Annie, putting down her knife and fork abruptly. "When you met *me*, then, Jenny, you thought *I* was a shocked survivor? So you and Alex have driven all that way to rescue me?"

There was a moment's awkward silence.

"Well, no, you couldn't really say that," said Alex, leaning forward earnestly. "I think what we find is that every time we learn of variations on our own brushes with relationship meltdown, it kind of rescues *us* a tiny bit. It's entirely selfish of us. I think we dread another bout of the disease. We have, after all, both made exactly the same mistake twice over. It's almost as if our Narcissist immune system, belatedly stoked up a bit, gets an extra boost every time we revise our own experience to make fresh deductions, or are lucky enough to chance upon the experience of others to learn from. It would appear to be a never ending process of recovery.

"So I suppose what we're asking is whether we can find out more about what you went through, Annie, for us to add it to our own First Aid kit, so to speak. And if you're interested in what we're talking about, Bianca, we would really appreciate hearing about what you've experienced, if it seems even the slightest bit relevant to all this stuff, from your point of view, and where you both are now with it all. I suppose that's why we're here. I admit it all sounds pretty daft, even to us."

"Especially to us!" laughed Jenny, a little nervously.

The other two women eyed one another questioningly for a moment. Bianca turned back to Alex.

"And do you intend to write about what you gather, to demonstrate variety of experience?" she asked lightly.

"Well, we haven't thought much about an end product, really," answered Alex. "We just carry on with investigating because there seems to be something constructive about the process itself. I'm not sure why that's so. We haven't found any one else among friends or family who is in any way intrigued by the whole exploration into Narcissism and dysfunctional relationships, and surviving the aftermath of it, and all that.

"You could say we're here because we're almost desperate for a bit of outside interest and encouragement, worried that we're just a couple of nutters who are sharing the same weird obsessions. Perhaps we both just 'need to get out more', including out of all this investigation! We don't know. We kind of wondered if you might know more."

She shrugged slightly, in a gesture of uncertainty. Jenny nodded, confirming the message of confusion with an uplift of her eyebrows. There was another pause.

"You go first, Annie."

Bianca spoke softly, and Annie nodded, with a slight intake of breath. Alex and Jenny felt an instant wave of relief, even before a word was spoken. They hadn't caused offence! These two women round this table were, amazingly enough, going to give them the benefit of the doubt. It was almost too good to be true, but it was true, nonetheless. Incredulity and elation surged through Alex and, for a brief moment, she found it hard to remain impassive. Jenny achieved apparent calm with more ease but she, too, felt instantly released from the tight grip of anxiety. They took up their turn as audience while Annie put down her napkin and cleared her throat.

"Well, – er – I suppose you could say that I was asking for trouble. I was employed by an organisation which supplied young women to serve male customers food, drink and pleasant distraction! We hated the term 'Trolley Dolly', as we were sometimes labelled back then, in the early Seventies, but actually all our training was about passengers feeling cherished as they were served; in particular, of course, the big spending, business class clients who were inevitably men, back in those days. So our so called sex appeal was a key factor in our employment. We were actually trained to apply makeup in a particular style, for a corporate image. It was odd that all of us girls, once we were in our uniforms and had painted on our required application of makeup, managed to end up looking mass produced. If you saw us as our ordinary selves, we'd look quite different from one another, although I suppose we were all tallish and slim, since that was the regulation build at that time, to get an air hostess job in the airlines.

"I was lucky because I was naturally thin, and found it easy to keep my weight steady but even for me, the monthly weigh ins were humiliating. I remember that some of us used to take handfuls of laxatives for a couple of days before getting on those awful scales, and we certainly did our best to come in at an ever decreasing weight. We'd remove watches and ear studs and even cut our toe nails or shave our legs at dawn on the dreaded scale hopping day. It's quite incredible, really, that we played along with the whole madness of it. But the pay seemed okay to us back then, and we all felt sort of privileged to have that job. You got a lot of sort of oohing and ahhhing about being an air hostess when you were off duty which was funny, but sort of good for the ego. Seems amazing, looking back on it now.

"So I guess we were encouraged to think of ourselves as society hostesses, in an old fashioned, classy sort of way. The term 'air hostess' probably struck us as really quite accurate for some of what we were trained to do on board the aircraft, although it left out the rushing about / skivvy part of the job, as well as all the safety training. We were definitely supposed to increase the glamour element of the journey for the male patrons of expensive trips. I suppose the theory was that if their sex drives were somehow engaged by our team of attentive air hostesses, they were expected to come back for more long haul flying with our airline because they'd remember the tingly, flattering effects on their egos, and forget the actual boring hours of the flight itself."

Annie paused at this point, glancing round the table as if to reassure herself that her listeners were with her. It was evident that they were, and she seemed momentarily discomforted by their attentive silence. She took a gulp of her wine and then put the glass back down on the table before taking up her narrative again.

"Well, amongst us girls, there really wasn't much cat fighting, or that sort of thing. You might think there must have been, but we really were quite supportive of one another most of the time. We weren't competitive about who was the most attractive or anything like that. I don't think any of us regarded male attention on flights as anything more than a regular feature of the job. Anyway, as I said, we were all done up to look more or less the same, and that meant we didn't really see ourselves as individuals when we were flying. As for our social life off duty, there wasn't much because the life style was so disruptive, and I think we were all mostly catching up on sleep or trying to work out where we were when we woke up! Having a serious boyfriend would have been very difficult but if you managed it, you were in danger of losing the job because back then, committed relationships were definitely a 'no no'.

"The one aspect of the job which could cause rivalry between us was to do with the pilots. If you got attention from one of them, that was quite something, I can tell you. And that's what happened to me. I should have knocked it on the head straight away, of course, but I was just bowled over by Dave right from the moment he laid a finger on me. He was a good looking Aussie in the first place, but in uniform he was just absolutely gorgeous! He was also funny and charming and extremely popular. Everyone in the airline rated him very highly as a pilot and as a great guy to have around.

"Well, of course, a bit of his attention focused on me, and I was smitten. I sort of knew he had a wife back in Australia, but there were no kids and he claimed they were already separated – they probably were. Anyway, one thing led to another very quickly, and I ended up using his Aussie flat as a base at times between flights, and he stayed with me in my flat in London as well, though all this had to be kept secret, of course.

"At the start it was all just incredible; I felt like I'd died and gone to heaven. It wasn't that I'd been unhappy before. I really loved where I lived. I was very lucky because I'd been able to do up my flat really well, through a trust my parents had set up for me which I could tap into once I was an adult. I was quite keen on the whole décor thing, and Dave really got a buzz from the sort of style I'd chosen for the place. He treated me like royalty, he really did. I was just perfect for him, he'd tell me; he didn't know such a wonderful woman could live on this earth; oh, I was just the best ever! He was always doing the most wonderfully romantic things for me, and taking my breath away. I could hardly believe I could be so important to a man of his quality, but apparently I was!

"We were both quite amazed at ourselves, I think. We were beginning to be the sort of Londoners who could carry it off somehow, although really we were just country stock, me from a terraced house in Cheshire originally, and him from some Outback group of tin shacks, brought up with no father and an under aged mother who went missing half the time, he told me on one occasion when he was very drunk. I'm not sure that was true. I do know that he was adopted by an older couple with no children themselves, in Sidney, soon after his real mum died. Anyway, I never found out whereabouts he was based originally. I don't think either of us was keen to let the other one into the world we actually came from.

"My family didn't even know about Dave's existence for years, and when we were in Sydney, I never saw him outside a five mile radius of our apartment, or met anyone from his past. He seemed to be estranged from his adoptive parents, but I don't know why. We were really quite isolated socially because of our jobs and the two bases at opposite sides of the world and the need to keep our relationship secret. But for a while there in London, we did kind of get drawn into an 'in crowd' where no questions were asked and we just must have looked the part, both of us. We had quite a ball, actually! That was all a very long time ago, of course."

Annie glanced round at her companions with a fleeting gesture directed at her own face. The slight whisper of self deprecating laughter was supportive all round, but Bianca seized the opportunity of this particular distraction to ask about further food ordering. All four women were soon scanning the limited choices available for a dessert which they might enjoy. Once the orders had been collected, Annie took up her story again, but more hurriedly than before, two slight frown lines creasing her brow just above the bridge of her nose.

"Well, it couldn't have lasted like that, really, burning the candle at both ends. Over a couple of years, some of Dave's charming attributes began to disappear, at least as far as I was concerned. He could still be utterly delightful with our friends and with new acquaintances, but somehow, I seemed to irritate him more and more, though, for the life of me, I couldn't understand what I was doing differently. Dave gradually began to get tetchy with me about all sorts of things but in particular, about my looks. He said I was beginning to – er – 'go off' was his phrase.

"About that time, I went down with glandular fever and was off work for quite a while. Dave really loathed me being ill. He simply couldn't see why I wasn't up and about within three days, and kept telling me there was nothing wrong with me. He began shouting all sorts of abuse at me, about what a lazy, useless cow I was; that would be on a good day, mind you, because he could express himself a lot more forcibly than that!

"My doctor advised me to consider a change of job; my parents did know about that, actually. They had been very keen that I should get out of the airline business and I think they were hoping I'd come up north again and settle nearer them. They wanted me to marry a local boy and have the standard two kids! They still knew nothing about Dave, of course.

"When I'd been flying, my mum was always watching the news for fear of air crashes, but now I suppose it made it just as bad for them that I'd become ill and they had been firmly discouraged from helping me recuperate or anything. Once I recovered, there'd be a rare fleeting visit I'd make back home, but that was difficult because I found it hard to lie to them about my life.

"Well, I was secretly in agreement with one part of their hopes for me. I wanted to fall pregnant, but it was Dave's baby I yearned for, and he wouldn't hear of it. Once I'd fully recovered from the glandular fever and wasn't working for the airline any more, I was job hunting in London, and Dave was often away, of course. It seemed to me he was staying longer in our Sydney apartment than he needed to each month, and that began to increase the rows between us. He said I was getting paranoid and I think maybe I was. I was certainly spending too much time hanging around the flat, feeling at a loose end.

"Things improved when I began doing private interior design work, and I remember Dave was really chuffed that one of the places I did was in Eaton Square. I didn't miss the air hostess job, and gradually, I began to find my own working connections, and made a few really good friends through commissions I undertook.

"I knew Dave was a difficult man but as far as I could see, dealing with demanding male expectations was pretty much what other women round me were doing, and the fact that he was away a lot gave me the freedom of pleasing myself most of the time, which I began to value. My friends said I was lucky that I had the best of both worlds, and I began to see that you could look at it like that. So I trained myself to be the perfect woman when he was back with me, and to run everything exactly as he wanted it. Things went a lot more smoothly then, for quite a while.

"But there was always this problem with me that I wanted a baby. I could do all the glamour underwear bit and all the sexy hanging from the chandelier type business that Dave wanted; it was fine by me. I could adjust how I looked and what I wore when he was around – step it up a bit – without any problem at all. I went very blonde, at that time, I remember, and it did appear to be the case that guys preferred blondes; I really experienced the accuracy of that, first hand! Believe it or not, I actually had a brunette wig custom made to look exactly like my hair was before. It cost hundreds! I reckoned that if I had to visit up north, I'd wear it and no questions would be asked. Never had the nerve to try it out, though. I simply didn't show up at home for a long time.

"During those years, I kept on at Dave about how I wanted a baby but he still wouldn't consider it. Once when I was overdue and thought I might be pregnant, he'd actually worked out himself that my period was late, and he went absolutely crazy. I think that may have been the first time he became physically violent with me, though he said he was sorry afterwards, and that it wouldn't happen again. It did, though, and more and more often.

"He never hurt my face, but he would force me down from behind until I was kneeling with my back to him, and then he would kick me more and more aggressively; 'booting the bitch' he'd call it. It would start as a sort of half jokey, punishment thing, as if it was a game. Sometimes he would suddenly stop, and be really sweet and gentle with me. But at other times, he seemed determined to continue until I collapsed. Anyway, I wasn't pregnant, that first time he did it, as it turned out. I did lose two pregnancies over the next three years, actually, and looking back on it, he knew my body's cycle so well that I think he might have meant to kick them out of me from the very start."

Annie sighed, glancing round briefly at her hushed audience. She was privately aware of her own childlessness and the fact that all her three listeners were mothers.

"Another thing that started to drive him crazy was if I seemed to being doing something new which I'd set up myself. He couldn't bear it when I began to study for an Interior Design qualification. He loathed me doing Screen Printing evening classes. Every change I made began to seem like a personal challenge to him, and the more I tried to adapt to his demands, the more new demands there were. He began saying there was something seriously wrong with me mentally. He had become interested in Psychology at this time and acquired a load of heavy text books. He made out that he was trying to diagnose what sort of paranoia I was suffering from. He used to say he'd get out of flying, take a degree in Psychology and then make a fortune out of over-privileged nutters like me.

"He'd hurl various psychological labels at me and he'd yell things like that I just played with the notion of pregnancy, but would never grow up enough to be a real mother. If I shouted back, things would get really nasty and he'd push me back into the wall with his foot wedged over mine, and threaten to burn bits of my hair off with his lighter. Even though he never did more than hold the lighter flame close to my face, I got really terrified of him after he started that stuff. I began to get the shakes quite often and he'd go even more nuts if he noticed I was trembling. It seemed to trigger off an attack of rage in him immediately. Often, he'd go into the kitchen and start smashing glasses and plates and anything he could lay his hands on. Funnily enough, he always only smashed up kitchen stuff, never the best china which he had selected in the first place. I guess he knew that the kitchen was my special place of safety, and that it was chaotic noise and destruction there which really got to me. I knew I had to get out."

Alex and Jenny were wide eyed as they listened. Bianca, although familiar with the denouement of Annie's story, was no less involved, shaking her head slightly as her friend was speaking, catching Jenny's glance as she did so.

"So basically, one month when I knew he'd be based in Sydney for at least three weeks, though it was creeping up to five or six weeks at a stretch, I planned it all out with the help of one very good friend nearby, and I just did a runner. I went back to Cheshire where I had my family and my good friends from school and gradually, I began to pull myself together. Dave traced me, of course, and there were some horrible confrontations by phone and letter, but he never actually came to my doorstep. I lived in terror that he would, for years.

"The London flat was in my name and he had never contributed towards the mortgage or the running costs; he had his own costs maintaining his base in Australia and I'd never paid towards those. It had always seemed to me that we shared our living expenses very fairly but after I left, he lied about our finances and claimed I'd shafted him. He threatened to sue me for every penny I'd got. It was all a nightmare, really."

Annie's head was lowered, but she spoke loudly enough to be heard.

"Anyway, he had a new woman in Australia, of course, and within a year, I heard that he had got divorced from his first wife so that he could marry her.

"The last thing I ever got from him was a photo sent through the post, about six years after I'd left. There was no letter inside and nothing written on the back of the snap. The picture was of Dave in a graduation gown, and he had one of those funny little mortar board hats with a tassel hanging down from it, perched on his head. He's looking at the camera and there's this sort of horrible leer on his face. In one arm he's holding a little boy with blond hair who is smiling round towards the camera. He looks about two years old, arms round his daddy's neck. Dave's other arm is stretched out towards the camera, but his hand is facing back towards his body with only his middle finger yanked up aggressively just to the other side of his face. He is posing directly for me. And it's a picture of Pure Hate."

There was a pause as the two listeners who were new to this last image tried to assimilate it.

"God!" whispered Alex. There was silence for a few moments, before all three listeners shook or lowered their heads, and there were communal murmurs about the 'sickness' of the described pose and its venomous message.

"Um – have you still got the photo?" asked Jenny tentatively.
"Yes, somewhere. Not sure where. Can't bear to look at it ever again, but somehow can't seek it out to destroy it, either. I suppose it might be useful to you for your research?"
Annie giggled slightly, though without a hint of a smile.
"It'd make a great front cover to a book about malignant Narcissists!" Jenny said, and they all laughed, glad of the relief.
"So that's the real end of my story, I suppose," commented Annie, picking up her dessert spoon for the first time. "Not very pleasant, is it? But you haven't heard anything yet! Wait until Bianca gets started; my tale's like a Sunday school picnic compared with hers."
Alex and Jenny glanced at one another momentarily, eyebrows raised. This had not been what they had expected. It had not occurred to either of them that there could be a league table of disordered partners and that their particular case studies might not in the Premier club at all, if they were being measured for devastation in their field. Alex shared this reflection with the others and there was some general chat about types of Domestic Violence and degrees of manipulation, power and control which might, or might not, fall short of actual pathology.
Bianca seemed in no hurry to present her own experiences, and there was some further delay which involved finishing desserts, ordering coffees and a couple of visits to the toilet-block beyond the side entrance of the pub before she eventually took up the theme which Annie had introduced for her.
"Well, I first got to know Andy when I was still at our local secondary school and he had only just left. We weren't quite childhood sweethearts but we were engaged by the time he was eighteen and me seventeen. Our families lived within two streets of each other in Bideford and it was the sort of community where we kids could play by roaming the streets in freedom and, apart from a bite of lunch, not be expected home before dark.
"Funny thing about running wild like that – it seemed to lose its appeal once we were teenagers. Back then, we girls seemed to be in an enormous hurry to go steady with just the one boy. Goodness knows why, but it was as if girls back then wanted to be like their mums as quickly as possible. Seems weird, really, with

so much freedom to roam, that we didn't go on to do any of that teenage crowd friendship thing which my own children did right up into their 20's.

"Anyway, I was sure that Andy was the one for me. We didn't have a penny between us but in the blink of an eye, there we were, man and wife, him window cleaning every hour God gave him when it wasn't lashing it down, and me working in the bank. We rented a damp, one bedroom flat, but it was paradise to us. I suppose maybe what we wanted most was privacy, far away from our nosey families and neighbours, and perhaps it was also about having the chance to have sex often without being caught at it and getting an earful about it, or getting 'a bun in the oven', and causing disgrace to the family.

"It wasn't long, though, before there was a legitimate bun in the oven, and by the time I was twenty eight, we had four youngsters and a tiny, three bedroom house which was bursting at the seams. Looking back, we seemed really happy then. Andy was a good dad and although we were still pretty strapped for cash, trying to pay the rent and manage on just the one salary, I had no worries about our marriage. Andy was careful with money and so was I, and he'd never been a drinker or a smoker.

"Actually, he absolutely loathed even the sight of cigarettes! He had lost his mum when he was only six, through lung cancer, and his family had had a dreadful time of it. His father had sunk into a terrible low after the loss of his wife, and Andy had had to look out for his two younger brothers and his dad, and he kind of lost his childhood because of that.

"Back then, I don't know if his dad had realised that it was his wife's heavy smoking habit that had given her such a prolonged and agonising death, but he was certainly very angry about losing her and just couldn't hold it together for his sons for quite a long time. I think he pulled it together again eventually, but he never remarried. His older sister came to live in the house with him later on, and I think she helped him to run the household.

"Anyway, at the time that I met him, Andy was devoted to his dad and was in close touch with his brothers, still keeping an eye on both of them! He was always the responsible one and that's what he prided himself on being. He was very sensible about everything.

That meant that he and I were doing all right as a couple, too; we never had rows about money, like other couples we knew. He wasn't a womaniser, either. If he was passionate about anything, it was about being a good provider for his family, and what more could you ask for than that?

"Well, time went on, and then Andy got a chance to set up business with a friend, carpet laying. It meant taking a risk but there seemed to be big money in wall to wall carpeting, back then, and his mate was already doing almost too well because he couldn't handle the orders on his own. So Andy and I discussed it, and we decided to go for it, and he never looked back. Don't get me wrong; it wasn't easy work! He was half crippled at first because he wasn't used to being cramped up on his knees for hours at a time and, to begin with, it nearly drove him round the bend. He missed the outdoor life of window cleaning, too, because he was always one for fresh air, was Andy. North Devon is a great place for wide open spaces and the river and beaches and all that, and I think he had always enjoyed being perched high up on the ladder, sometimes able to look out over the trees to the horizon.

"Well, the carpet business expanded, and by the time our kids were all at secondary school, we were 'upwardly mobile', I suppose the term is now. Andy wasn't on his knees anymore; oh no! He was running 'Magic Carpets' outlets all over the county and, later on, over most of the South of England. I didn't need to work any longer, and could be at home for the kids. We had a really lovely home, too, all paid for, and a lifestyle we'd never dreamed of when we first got together. You'd have thought we'd have counted our blessings but somehow, things began to go wrong, though it was only gradually at first.

"We had some trouble with our eldest boy – truanting, smoking, you know, the normal teenager business and nothing major – but Andy took it very hard. He seemed to want us to be the Perfect Family and he just couldn't get his head round it if anything happened to fracture that image the slightest bit. Neither of us came from that sort of set up and I really can't tell you where he got that idea from. He seemed to think that because our children were having the sort of rich kid life that we never had, they ought to have higher standards of behaviour than us lot ever did as youngsters. The other three never gave us any problems, and Stephen, the eldest, cleaned up his act in his early 20's and is a Senior Social worker now, totally dedicated to the job!

"Looking back on those far off times, I think now that Andy was probably depressed, but there was nothing obviously the matter physically with him, and the business was still doing great! We were beginning to take regular family holidays abroad and we even got a sauna built at the back of the house; oh, we had it all! But he and I weren't getting on too well by this time.

"We were hardly speaking, really, because he always seemed absolutely bowed down by the business; he couldn't think about anything else. Those family holidays! After the third one, he wouldn't come with us himself, but he'd pay for my sister to come along with her family. And to tell you the truth, we all had a better time without him. So we didn't object.

"I think it was around about then that he started giving me the odd shove if we had words, but maybe he had done it when the kids were smaller. I'm not sure. Anyway, it began to get worse. I never wanted the kids to know anything about it. So if he hit me, I'd never shout or hit back or anything; I'd get away fast and try to forget it. It got harder to do that when he started to leave marks on me. He would occasionally get me round the neck and knock my head against the wall and that might leave thumb bruises round here…" Bianca indicated two points on either side of her neck.

"Anyway, I had the best collection of silk polo necks in town, I can tell you – every colour you can think of – and for a long time, I convinced myself that nobody knew. I was desperate to hide it. I was somehow very ashamed of those marks and what they said about us, despite our double garage and all our fancy finery.

"I suppose I believed that he'd change or I'd at least get better at avoiding situations which ended up in any sort of violence, but nothing I tried could prevent it from escalating. One time when I had to get myself to Out patients' because I thought my arm was fractured, I remember feeling ashamed that I could lie so convincingly in Casualty about what had happened, without even needing to plan out what I was going to say. When I got back in from the hospital – our youngest had left home by this time – Andy wasn't back from work and I sat there on my own in the kitchen, dreading what he would say when he got home, saw the plaster and realised that someone medical must have officially treated the break. But I remember when he did get back very late, and set eyes on the sling, he just broke down and wept. He swore it would never happen again; he was absolutely beside himself.

"It didn't stop, of course, though the pattern changed a bit. The violence didn't happen as often but when it did, it was worse, and immediately afterwards, Andy'd became more and more desperately upset. He'd sometimes start this terrible low howling, kind of like an injured animal; honestly, it'd freeze your blood. I knew something had gone wrong with him mentally, but he refused point blank to consider going to a doctor. He seemed to be getting some very weird obsessions. He had got some really strange idea into his head about an older couple in the neighbourhood spreading malicious rumours about him. These people weren't any trouble at all to us but were just a bit stand offish, maybe.

"Much worse than that, though, was that he began to rant on about this notion that Stephen, our eldest, wasn't his. There had never been any worries about that when I was first pregnant. In a small, close knit community like ours, childhood sweethearts knew everything there is to know about each other, you know, including exactly how many fillings they'd ever had in their teeth! It wasn't as if we'd had to get married or anything, although with baby Stephen arriving just ten months after the wedding, I imagine there was some finger counting locally, just to be sure! Everyone said Stephen was the spitting image of his dad, and he still is. There was never any question about Andy being all the kids' dad when they were young, but now it was as if Andy needed to destroy anything that meant something to him or me personally, and that included smashing up a happy family life for all of us.

"At least Andy didn't let on his doubts to Stephen himself, but he became more and more obsessed with using the idea against me as time went on. There was nothing I could say or do to convince him that Stephen was his child. I suggested more than once that he arranged medical testing privately, to prove it to him, but for various reasons, he would never agree to that. One explanation he gave was that it would hurt Stephen too much to find out he was a bastard. Actually, I think yes, Stephen would have been devastated to learn about his dad's doubts, but he would have been up for the test if it took me out of the firing line by proving Andy *was* his dad, which was dead obvious to everyone else. But I knew that then Andy would just have started questioning the paternity of one of the other three, because he was beginning to suggest I had been sleeping around since the marriage as well. I got called all the names under the sun when he had lost it – 'slut', 'slag', 'whore', 'town bike', and you wouldn't believe the things he accused me of when my sister and I and the kids had been on those holidays abroad, and he'd been back home.

"During this time, my youngest boy was back home living with us for a while, and he really did everything he could to help his dad and me. He didn't hear any of our rows, I don't think, and that must have meant that I put a good face on things, and Andy was obviously controlling himself as well. But anyway, Frank could sense an atmosphere all right, and he was deeply anxious about his dad's stress levels at work, and used to fret with me about it. He and his dad had been thick as thieves when he was a young lad, football fans together, and Andy was still his hero. It was the same with all the kids. Each and every one of them would have done anything for their dad. Frank thought Andy was depressed from being managing director; he felt it wasn't what he was cut out for at all. He reckoned that Andy needed to sell the business, rest on the fruits of his labours, and then begin to get back to enjoying the outdoor life of his youth; not window cleaning, of course, but maybe taking up golf or gliding or anything to get him outdoors again.

"But there was no talking to Andy about changing anything to do with his work-load because the company was employing over forty people by now, and he felt it was all down to him to keep the profits soaring. He wasn't one of life's delegators, our Andy!

"I can't tell you why I didn't take the initiative myself to get myself out of the firing line, or tell anyone what was really going on behind closed doors. If I'd have told Frank, he wouldn't have overreacted. He was a sensible lad and he would have worked on it with me, and we would have considered how and where to ask for help. He would have been supportive with both of us, and I know the whole family would have stood together. But I just couldn't bear them to find out about the violence because – because – well – maybe it was my pride or something. Anyway, I never told Frank.

"Once Frank moved out again, Andy occasionally took to smashing windows at night, in any room where he might find me hiding away from him. There'd be glass everywhere – sometimes in my hair, if I didn't move away quick enough. By now, he was constantly on about me trapping him into marriage and then expecting him to support one bastard son and even the next and the next one after that – were any of them his?

"Oddly enough, though, he never brought Rosie into these accusations, despite the fact that she was the only one of the four who took after my side of the family in looks, not his. There was no reasoning with him at all once he was out of control. The only way he seemed to be able to short circuit his fury was if he broke a window pane hard enough to make the glass come crashing down all around him.

"I got pretty handy at replacing window panes, using sprigs and putty, and making a nice job of it. But if Andy had smashed a bigger section of glass, I'd be in difficulties. I had to choose a different glazier every time to fix it up. I couldn't explain it happening almost every year when there were no ball parks anywhere near us, and absolutely no hint of vandalism in that upper crust part of the town. I think, by now, I had some sort of hostage mentality or something. I had become so frightened of Andy's outbursts that every minute of my life was built round appeasing him. That stage went on for a very long time.

"And then, one day, I'd had enough. It was exactly like it was for Annie. I just walked out. I went to a Women's Support Centre in Barnstaple for a short while, but no one in the family knew that. The next months that followed are a bit of a fog. The kids were all very concerned and my daughter was my rock. I went to stay with her. She had always adored her dad, but she was just as much there for me. They all thought I'd had some sort of nervous breakdown.

"Anyway, to cut a long story short, Andy and I were divorced within two years. The house was sold and he moved into an even bigger one ten miles away. Lord knows why, he had no need of it.

"In time, though, he got it together with a divorced woman who had two teenage girls, and then I suppose all that space was useful. He never tried to contact me or the boys once all the legal stuff was completed, but Rosie did keep in touch with him, and he would see her from time to time. He never let up on the job; worked himself to the ground and dropped dead from a massive heart attack when he was fifty one.

"Didn't leave a penny to any of his own kids – not even to Rosie. Left everything to the two step daughters. The will was explicit on that; devastatingly so. He provided for their mother for the rest of her life but those girls, who'd only been in his life a couple of years, were actually left more than three million pounds between them. It broke my children's hearts, not because of the money, but the fact that the will made it so very clear that he had deliberately disowned his first four children for no reason that any of us could fathom. We never talk about it anymore in the family. It's just too painful to bear."

She nodded round the table, blinking rather sharply. Annie turned to Alex and Jenny.

"See what I mean?" she asked softly.

Jenny made a hand gesture which could be interpreted as, "You've both been through hell." Alex sighed in agreement, eyes down. There was a pause before she raised her head and looked towards the two friends.

"Well, thank you. Thank you so much for letting us in on all that. I don't know – I don't know what to say. What you've both been through......! The one thing – er – that I can be sure of is that if, one day, in the future, we were ever to write up anything either of you have told us, we'd consult you both first. I mean, could we use any part of either story, if it came up?"

"Oh yes, of course! You'd alter the odd detail here and there, wouldn't you? And you wouldn't identify us by name at all. And anyway, we're talking about lifetimes long ago. We're both safe in different worlds now, aren't we, Annie? Perhaps in the recounting of it, we tend to get thrown back in there for a little while, but as we emerge, we realise how far we've come. Use whatever you'd like! After you wrote to Annie, we talked about what you might want, and we agreed we'd be okay if you ever chose to write up anything we told you. We're both really up for the idea of some sort of a book about all this. It'd be great, even if it only helped one person get out of a dangerous relationship quicker than we did."

Alex and Jenny gazed across at Bianca with delighted grins. She carried on, her voice becoming more advisory in tone.

"But I do think you'll need to balance it with at least one story where it works the other way round. You know, where it's a man under the power of a female, or female persecuting a woman, for that matter. And of course, Domestic Violence can easily be woman on man; you might present a case of that. Or what about disordered daughter on father, or sister on brother?

"You don't want to suggest that all men are bastards, after all, or that this sort of thing only happens in so called romantic partnerships. You said you are happily married to a good man, Alex, and I am now, too. I expect all four of us knew or know good men we could have lived with happily enough but chose not to for some reason or other, or maybe never got the chance to.

"And it's also important to consider the effect it has on boys and girls to be brought up by a damagingly domineering parent or grandparent or to be under the power of a pathologically controlling teacher or whatever. The damage done to the victim may be different according to the age and stage and the type of power being used, but it's certainly not confined to a broken heart or a broken body. Many survivors often don't even recognise the long term harm that has been done to them, as you were saying earlier. If that's the case, it's impossible for them ever to recover, isn't it? They won't even know what they've lost."

Bianca seemed to be warming to the theme of what should be investigated, especially as both Alex and Jenny were nodding enthusiastically, keen for her to continue.

"And if you're going to look at those sorts of variations, there's the point that in harmfully controlling relationships between two consenting adults, the victim has usually had some choice about engaging in the bonding in the first place, whereas an offspring or sibling hasn't. Sometimes the relationship might be about two controllers cornering their own little power domains and one becomes as bad as the other, even if it wasn't that way to begin with. Think of murdering partnerships like Hindley and Brady, or Fred and Rosemary West! And what about Blair and Bush? You'll have to decide on the scope of damaging behaviours you want to investigate and whether you are going to talk about 'Narcissists', and examine them as if they are a breed apart. After all, we all can put on an act, can't we, and suppress our feelings for others as a natural defence strategy, at times?"

Alex nodded, pleased to be confirmed in her own perplexities about handling the topic.

"Yes, we've agonised about some of those points already," she replied eagerly, "especially about the fact that neither of us have any qualification whatsoever, which could back up our scanty knowledge of any of this. Even the term 'Narcissist'; I mean, you could argue that it is meaningless on its own like that, since there are so many ways to interpret it, ranging from someone who uses the mirror rather too frequently to someone with a pathological Disorder of the Self. I shouldn't think we'll ever resolve those sorts of issues, and we'll end up with a lot of scruffy notes and nothing else to show for it. But it doesn't really matter, does it, if the process of doing it has started to clear our heads? That's what all this is really about, isn't it? The rehabilitation of the survivor!"

"But I want to know whether men like we've been describing could ever change and stop being controlling in that way?"

Annie was speaking now, earnest and intense in her questioning. "Is there medication which could deal with the symptoms, or long term therapy which might heal abusers? I understand that they can't be helped from within the relationship they are controlling but is there any other way they can get better?" She was looking upset. "After all, we keep talking about how we have to restore ourselves, but surely it's *them* who need to be different. Why blame the victim?"

"Well, from what I've read, some exploitative people mellow as they get older, but then I've also read in other books that as they get less attractive and powerful, their frustration mounts and they become worse." Alex was attempting to sound like an informed yet impartial observer at this point. "One reason why they may be considered less dangerous to others could be because, during the course of their lives, everyone in their orbit has finally learnt to stop trying to relate to them personally.

"Another possibility is that the early symptoms of dementia sometimes involve a breaking down of defences which can, in turn, reveal glimpses of a more open sort of connection. I think I read somewhere that Enid Blyton's younger daughter found her overbearing mother somewhat more approachable as her early onset dementia began to dismantle her pathological need for control."

Alex's words were beginning to take on a hint of authority. It was a tone which Jenny recognised immediately, as Alex continued to speak, glancing at Annie sympathetically.

"I don't think antidepressants help Narcissists to tune in to other people any better, from what I've read, and antipsychotic medication isn't really relevant because, as far as I know, they rarely hear Voices or see aliens in their soup. I'm afraid that part of their condition is a failure to recognise any need for treatment at all, since they often see other people as the problem, not them. Why seek to change if they are perfectly okay as they are? If they truly recognised that their stuck defences were standing in the way of genuine intimacy with others, I suspect they wouldn't be very far along the Narcissistic Disorder spectrum in the first place."

"So if they won't, or can't, change," added Jenny, concerned that Annie had not yet received a direct reply, "then the other person in the controlling relationship must, in order not to be brought down with them. It's not really about blaming the victim, actually; it's about the victim changing him or herself into a survivor. Some people seem to have a natural immunity to dysfunctional controllers. If we here have all been victims, there's a case for saying we need to develop that sort of immunity ourselves. Actually, it's how to do that which interests Alex and me the most.

"There doesn't seem to be much progress if all we do is fear other human beings in general and men in particular, but we obviously need to be on our guard. Quite a dilemma, really! Not much has been written about it, though there's lots and lots out there about Narcissistic traits and operational tactics. I suppose the recovery of the survivors is less interesting, medically. There's a sort of glamour, somehow, about pathological Narcissism which even seems to extend to those who are experts on it."

Annie still looked troubled and Bianca stretched forward a little towards her as she smiled round the table, subtly suggesting by this gesture that they might bring the discussion to a close. She endorsed the insinuation with a quietly spoken observation.

"I think we should get the bill now, if that's okay, and rely on our kind chauffeur to take us home. I have a grotty back, and sitting here much longer will cause it to flare up again. But all this has been absolutely fascinating and has given us so much to think about........"

"Yes, and I need to get back for Carla," added Annie, reaching into her handbag for the car keys.

All four women joined in the general round of supportive comments which followed, and the warmth between them did not dissipate as the bill was paid and they emerged from the now quite empty pub into the dark street outside. During the short return car journey, Jenny and Alex both felt equally relieved by the outcome of an evening which had seemed such an uncertain proposition beforehand. Once outside her house, Bianca levered herself gingerly out of the front seat and then turned to bid fond farewells to the passengers in the rear, before thanking Annie with a quick pat of her hand.

It wasn't long before Annie had also bid her guests good night and they had left her downstairs to 'see to a few things for Carla', while they sought the refuge of their bedroom. As soon as Jenny had closed their door, she turned toward Alex and they stood opposite one another, each poised to register the other's response.

"Phew!" breathed Alex.

Jenny lowered her head and patted the sides of her brow with flat palms, in an equivalent gesture of relief.

"Well, who'd ever, ever have guessed our great rescue mission would turn out like that!" she exclaimed, glancing up again towards Alex, after sitting down abruptly on her bed.

She continued incredulously, "In lots of ways, they rescued us, didn't they? They gave us a completely new way of understanding our men. All four of ours are really only garden-variety Narcissists when we compare them with their wilder infestations! And as for helping Annie, she didn't need us our services, anyway! I had no idea when we first spoke that she had a neighbour and friend of Bianca's quality, who was absolutely with her in all this stuff! And they were both so ready to tell us about it all, when really we were just two strangers bursting in on their lives from darkest Hampshire. It's amazing!"

"The relief!" intoned Alex, sitting down on the opposite bed and looking around vaguely for her sponge bag, before temporarily abandoning the search. "We were just so lucky that it worked out like this; mission sort of quietly aborted, instead of crash landing on the wrong side of the moon!"

Their bedtime preparations eventually performed, both women edged themselves gingerly into their starched linen, almost afraid to dislodge the perfection of the bed covers. There was no need for bedside lamps since neither woman wanted to read, but neither of them expected that sleep would be easily attainable. So they both lay in the darkness, shifting positions in their unfamiliar single beds and reshaping their huge, bulky pillows to a lower level of neck support until eventually, each of them found her own pathway to fragmented dreams.

CHAPTER 10

Departure Day

It was much to their surprise, the following morning, that they entered the kitchen at the appointed time and found Bianca at the kitchen table, sharing a coffee with the proprietor. Annie immediately rose as they came in, indicated their set places at the large pine table, and itemised their choices to eat and drink, almost officious in her demonstration of carrying out the second 'B' in her B and B contract.

In contrast, Bianca laughed up at them apologetically, waving them towards her as they approached their seats. "You see, I can't get enough of you two!" she joked. "Please forgive my intrusion but during the night my mind was chugging away, and I couldn't resist another bite of the cherry. So I popped round here to join you over breakfast. Is that all right?"

"Much more than all right!" exclaimed Alex warmly. Jenny echoed the sentiment as they drew back the chairs to sit opposite and beside her. All three of them were soon involved in a conversation along much the same lines as the night before, but there was a sort of unspoken agreement that it was lighter in tone while Annie was unable to join them round the table. Neither Jenny nor Alex was surprised to find that, even though they were sticking to cereal, toast and coffee, the breakfast fare was still lavish and the selection almost impossibly wide. Eventually, Annie was able to take her place with them and be assured that every possible whim of her guests had been indulged in full. By this time, Bianca was just taking up the theme of men, and how they cope with controlling women.

"Could you imagine two men collaborating together on the sort of research crusade that you two have launched?" she asked her audience, with a smile. "Suppose two husbands got together after their wives who were sisters, say, had both abruptly deserted their respective families in the space of a couple of years. Would the abandoned men meet to support one another, and try to work out how and why it had happened? Let's say that the husbands both knew there was something in the sisters' family history; I don't know...... well, something like, if the father had had a long term hidden relationship with another woman, or there was some awful secret about some grisly events which might have happened long ago in the woodshed. D'you think the husbands would work together to try to fathom out whether that family history could have influenced both their wives to bolt?"

Alex was quick to offer an answer.

"No, I don't think men would – not most men, anyway. My limited experience of deserted men is that they are extremely angry. Dan was quietly enraged with his departing wife when I first met him and his little Bella in London. It's my theory that she had upped and left without much warning because she felt sidelined by the loving warmth between Dan and Bella.

"Perhaps if he had understood that at the time, he would have been less bitter, and might have realised that her leaving was more to do with her insecurities about young motherhood than a rejection of him. But often, men seem to be unwilling to ferret any deeper down into their own emotions than the anger level. I suppose registering their deep sadness and loss might be too much for them to bear? So they move from anger to quiet bitterness and then to shutting the whole experience up in a box. I think they'd avoid analysing it with anyone, even a brother-in-law who was in the same boat."

"And why is that?" asked Jenny. "Is that just how most men are wired? For the survival of their genes down into the next generations, do they *have* to go out and do their propagating stuff, and leave the feely, fluffy stuff to the female, rearing the young?"

Jenny paused, and then continued to investigate this line of enquiry, trying to recall whatever she could about the selfish gene.

"The fact that men's sex drive is generally stronger than women's could be a wiring matter too, couldn't it? Wasn't there some research which showed that men think about having sex very much more often than women do? Nature doesn't go for monogamy within a restricted gene pool, after all. If the males put it about a bit, then there's more chance of an advantageous variant showing up in the next generation, and then future generations will gain further ground from those beneficial variants, as time goes on. Isn't that – um, roughly speaking, of course – what Darwin's theory of evolution is all about?"

"But we aren't just slaves to our wiring, surely?" commented Annie, in response. " I mean, I know that our hormones affect our moods, and our genes determine lots about us, but that doesn't mean that if we're an angry sort of person, wired to be an aggressive hunter and sexual predator, it's perfectly all right in this day and age to go around regarding other human beings as prey."

"Um ... well, I suppose there are a lot of different factors that make us act in certain ways in challenging environments," Jenny replied. "What exactly that action might be – rescuing a drowning child in fierce flood waters or beating up a pensioner who complains about the nightly drunken din outside his home – is obviously the essential question, Annie, as you say. The most super charged active person still has to choose how to use her or his driving energy to the benefit of others, or, at the least, how to do no unnecessary harm."

"Yes," nodded Bianca thoughtfully. "But might it be true to say that the majority of men, wired to hunt and attack in the context of a brutal struggle for survival, are less likely than women to spend time sorting out feelings more complex than Flight or Fight?"

She was leaning forward in her chair, elbows on the table. "The interesting thing," she reflected, "is that men are apparently less prone to depression than women, aren't they? So maybe it's actually healthier not to analyse things and become obsessed with trying to understand the feelings which get tangled up in our close relationships? Do many women go to the opposite extreme and get themselves so bogged down in obsessive thinking that they then become incapable of Flight or Fight and just freeze themselves into immobility? Depression is a sort of frozen state, isn't it? I'm talking about the sort of depression which is a psychological response to experience, not the result of a chemical hiatus in the brain."

"Well, I think I'd rather be frozen stiff than be a serial killer," remarked Annie. "Maybe neither of them count as emotionally healthy, but at least with depression, we are turning the destruction in on ourselves, not executing innocent victims because somehow they pressed our buttons without the slightest inkling of the danger."

"Actually, I do believe that reactive depression can be beneficial to some extent; it can contain a restorative element within it. I think maybe its potential benefit to the sufferer is usually lost under the automatic presumption of disease." Alex nodded towards Annie, in agreement. "We are so afraid of it, but maybe it is partially a case of our intuition telling us to Play Possum and act dead for a while, which may be far wiser than Flight or Fight in some cases.

"If we could only be grateful for the Fog and the Bewilderment, maybe it would clear more quickly because it would have served its protective purpose in the crisis and could then dissipate naturally, in its own good time. But as it is, we are so horrified to find ourselves immobilised and in need of treatment that we are ashamed and mad at ourselves. That shame darkens the Fog around us and makes what might be an innate protection a suffocating disability instead.

"However, I'm not sure that it's right to say that men use instant Flight or Fight responses more than women do. Perhaps more men 'freeze' into depression than we realise but maybe they themselves just don't recognise it. I think it confuses matters that men are less likely than women to go to the doctor, even if they suspect that something's wrong in their heads. They are often afraid to be laid off work because not to be able to work effectively hits at their sense of identity as a provider. Or they may consider that because they have no obvious physical ailment, they are bound to come across as work–shy malingerers. So depression in men will probably often go undiagnosed. That's a cultural thing, I suppose, that men are reluctant to seek help, in case they appear pathetic, don't you think? It seems to me that women are more likely to seek support from friends and family, and to consult each other and their doctor if it eventually appears necessary, without feeling so shamed up about a troubled mind."

Alex paused, uncertain if the others were following her. Reassured that they were, she tried to relate what she was saying to both Annie and Bianca's comments.

"Chemical stuff may come into it. I don't know much about it but I think depleted levels of serotonin and testosterone make depression more likely, while high levels of cortisol help us to survive stressful emergencies. Apparently, it isn't true that people with high levels of testosterone are necessarily more aggressive than those with average levels, although they have more energy and might be more apt to take risks. We used to think men were more likely to be aggressive than women because of their hormonal systems, but I think it's all far more complex than that.

"There are certainly women who are brilliant at dominating men aggressively to the point that the men are virtually their puppets. That series 'The Sopranos' on tele; did you ever see it? It was about –um- sort of Mafia families and their private lives and there was lots of killing going on, but at the very heart of all the violence was a little ol' matriarch who manipulated the gang warfare within and beyond the family out of her own pathological need for power and control. Yet the dear wee grandma herself never fired a shot. So maybe it doesn't really help us much to try to sort out who does what along gender lines. It seems to me that lots of it boils down to environment and the socialisation process, from the very earliest weeks of life; maybe even before birth itself."

"So it's all the mother's fault, then? Surely we are laying the blame on women again, here?" Annie sounded indignant.

"No, not really. Parents who rear their children in a partnership will both present a role model for interaction with the opposite sex, although they will probably be as unaware of this as their children are. It's obviously helpful if the couple has a healthy relationship, but if it's a seriously unhealthy one, the children are likely to grow up confusing abuse with love. Boys may unconsciously seek a controlling woman when they grow up because they saw their father driven into forlorn passivity under the direction of their manipulative mother. Or girls may be totally unaware that they are seeking to replicate a relationship between a bullying father and a compliant mother from the previous generation, or even the one before that.

"An abusive pairing is very unlikely to provide a healthy environment for a new baby, but I can't see why responsibility for child rearing should rest on the female of the partnership more than the male. How mothers, and any other caregivers, for that matter, interact with each other and with their babies is influenced in all sorts of complex ways by the society in which they are living, and that may well be a divided, exploitative society where dominant male expectations generally win out, at least as far as male offspring are concerned."

Alex paused, trying to sound a bit more tentative as she continued, "I think there could be an important point to be made here about child rearing and gender. Um – it's pretty obvious that most infant girls are initially reared by a female primary caregiver. When these little girls grow up, they won't usually have strong unconscious patterning, based on their own personal experience from their earliest stages of life, of potential close nurturing from a *male*.

"Infants of either sex generally receive considerably more of their earliest physical and emotional nurturing – their nutrition and their cuddling – from the female parent than from the male. Girls reared within a healthy family dynamic might therefore grow up to be fairly open-minded about how a mutually supportive, intimate partnership with a man could work in their adult family of choice, because it's long been unfamiliar territory for them. I admit that girls may experience a pervasive social patterning based round romantic pop songs and Happy Ever After fiction, of course, but that may have less impact because it kicks in rather later.

"For a man, it must be different, mustn't it? He's extremely likely to have been raised at the earliest stages of life mainly by his mother. And all his early supervisors and authority figures – his nursery and primary teachers and babysitters – are also likely to be female. A particular style of long term female care and control may become a strong pattern which boys subconsciously seek to repeat in their own chosen adult relationship with women later on. Even if the family dynamic he experienced was of mutual warmth and respect between his parents, that unconscious drive for repetition would mean that the subsequent power balance between the man and any chosen female partner of his is very unlikely to have been actively considered and mutually negotiated between the couple, over time.

"So – how's this for a theory, folks? Could it be that men who choose women partners are even more likely to fall into a role of being dominated by a controller than women who choose men partners are? Consider the interesting fact that some men go out and pay good money to put themselves into the hands of Dominatrix women who provide experiences associated with infant eroticism by – well, I don't know what the service involves, but I think it's about stimulating basic bodily functions. I don't know any statistics, but I'd be surprised if as many women want to experience a similar domination of – say – their anal functioning through the services of a paid man."

"I'm losing the thread of this," commented Jenny anxiously. "What point are you making here, Alex?"

"Well, I suppose what I'm saying is that women and men may both be just as likely to seek to establish control over the other in a relationship. The point I am making – probably ineptly, I have to say! – is that females are not actually primed to expect a pattern of constant male domination which was deeply engrained within them from their very first moments of life.

"So if women begin to realise that their Self is subtly under attack somehow, they are profoundly shocked. They didn't experience physical and emotional dependence on a member of the opposite sex from their earliest existence in the way their brothers did. By way of contrast, many a decent man just resigns himself, in adulthood, to yet another power-wielding female, and tries to play the 'good boy' in response, for a quiet life."

Bianca nodded, running her fingers through her hair. "I think our society is becoming more and more alert to the danger from men who obviously aren't in the least resigned to dependency on women and are, instead, pathologically resentful of it. That sort of male resentment could sometimes be unconsciously grounded on female abuse of power from way back couldn't it?

"Girls and women who suffer emotional or physical violence in their relationships are now generally acknowledged to be at terrible risk of profound damage and even death, but it's probably less acknowledged that female mistreatment of boys and men can also have left a trail of devastation in its wake.

"The damage done in a disordered mother – son relationship may blight the lad's life, but any women who later seek to relate to him once he's an adult may also end up wounded by what went on between mother and dependent son, many years before, and is still operating from somewhere deeply buried in the man's psyche.

"I've good reason to be relieved that Domestic Violence or Abuse (male on female) has, thank God, become a major issue in society now. The result is that many women, even teenage or younger, might at least come to recognise that male abuse of them is a violation of their rights. They may have a chance of getting themselves out of abusive relationships, supposing that they can access some sort of supportive network to help them.

"But perhaps you're right, Alex. It may well be that a lot of men can't even recognise subjection to the female of the species because they were dependent on a woman for survival from the moment they took their first breath, and even before that, of course, for the nine months in the womb. I admit that for the majority of all babies, this dependence may be safe enough, but we can't expect all mothers to use their power over infants and toddlers with good enough levels of compassion. After all, their mothering skills will inevitably reflect those of their own parents, and that could have been a very negative influence – you know, 'Children should be seen but not heard' sort of stuff, or much worse.

"And, as well as that, the pressures of parenting, such as sleep deprivation and social isolation and just sheer economic hardship can be pretty awful. When the chips are tumbling down, of course, it's the woman who is most likely to be the one left holding the babies. For example, that's what happened to both of you, wasn't it? Your husbands sailed off and there you were; two kids apiece." Bianca tilted her head towards Jenny and Alex sympathetically. Alex glanced back at her with a nod and a smile before taking the topic further herself.

"Another complication, I think, arises from breast feeding. The relationship between an infant daughter and her father surely can't involve the same sort of complex two way sensual bonding as a male child feeding at his mother's breast? Even in today's bottle-fed culture, that sucking process while the boy infant is being wedged close to the female's upper body must be a naturally erotic experience, mustn't it?

"Our society certainly seems to send out overtly erotic messages about women's breasts, mainly as they are perceived by men. One of many possible results of this is that you get some new fathers who have considerable difficulties accepting the sight of their infant son nestled within those breasts which the husband considered his territorial play centre! And some women, of course, never quite release their male offspring from that extraordinarily intimate physical bond of feeding at the breast. So perhaps, for all sorts of complex reasons, there is an ambiguity in men's perception of women as providers of nourishment and pleasure, but also as enforcers of painful restrictions.

"If boys enter subsequent adult relationships still unconsciously confused about what is loving mutuality and what is dominating control, they will tend to adapt to whatever they get from their female partner, without spotting a cause for complaint. After all, the domination men suffer at the hands of women is less likely to be evident in terms of physical threat or superior fist force. If there's any sexual abuse, female on male, the callous invasion on the partner's sexual territory will usually involve psychological warfare rather than sheer brute force and urgently functional hydraulics.

"I can't really see how a woman could use her undercarriage equipment to rape a man, although she can undoubtedly entice involuntary responses in him. It must surely be a considerable disadvantage to a man that his genitals are all too exposed to assessment and ridicule by an abusive partner. Presumably, that can be as damaging to the man's sense of Self as male on female sexual abuse, but it is probably less acknowledged as such by our society.

"Men's physical abuse of females is much more widely recognised and condemned than vice versa. I know for a fact that some people consider it good luck for little boys if they got a bit of abusive slap and tickle from an attractive female teenage baby sitter, whereas the same people would be enraged if a little girl was similarly sneakily molested by a teenage boy."

"We don't really take it on board that a female can be an abuser; is that what you mean?" asked Jenny, still attempting to keep the thread of Alex's argument clear in her mind.

"Yes, that's roughly what I'm on about. We have to believe that mothers, with their inordinate power over our life and death when we are tiny and completely vulnerable, must have wished us well, if we have survived to tell the tale!

"Perhaps men won't get depressed or fogged up or bewildered, even if every aspect of their adult relationship is being manipulated by their women, because they won't usually even catch on to it. After all, the luckier little chaps may have been very sweetly conditioned by the main female caregivers of their early childhood *not* to catch on to it: 'Oh you clever boy! You've done a beautiful poo poo in the pot all by yourself – aren't you a genius!' sort of thing. What the mother actually feels is huge relief that she might be able to stop clearing up shit pretty soon, but she's not going to be straight about expressing that!

"So the infant grows into a boy who grows into a man, totally unaware that his jubilant pleasure at his daily poo procedures is actually a response deeply conditioned within him by his flatteringly persuasive mother.

"As far as I can see, men don't usually bother to analyse why they feel proud or ashamed about anything. They aren't likely to explore any such personal responses with their closest mates, as women might well do, in the company of other women. Men often keep the workings of their relationships with women in soft focus while their sharpened perception is directed towards the world of professional achievement.

"And.... if ever men do voice a suspicion of subterfuge, a skilful female partner can make mincemeat of their fumbling unease in no time. The pacified men will then usually just roll over, paws up. Or maybe they'll compartmentalise it, and be Mr. Masterful at work, but a lapdog at home. You could say that some men unconsciously expect and seek to be dominated in that way by women. After all, we crave the familiar, don't we? But that doesn't let women off the hook for being abusive controllers in their intimate relationships. They just happen to get away with it because a lot of sons are conditioned eventually to give their intimate woman partner, their chosen mother substitute, the benefit of the doubt."

"Gosh, Alex – that all sounds terribly clever, but I thought we were trying to achieve some sort of damage limitation on what men controllers have done to us. And now you're saying that women may actually be the original controllers all along. What happened to us four women then?" Annie seemed perplexed.

"May I answer that?" interposed Bianca quickly. "It seems to me that being prepared to believe the best of women (or of men, for that matter) might actually be a healthy position, until the individual we are close to gives us reason to question our trust and safety. We'll probably be able to weigh up the threat effectively if we look carefully at our own intuitive response to the person; the clues will all be there in our inner reaction to him or her. So although we are vulnerable when we give the opposite sex the benefit of the doubt, it's not necessarily signing away our own rights. We simply have to be very aware, in the here and now, of our responses in our gut. That's our best guide, really, as to where to put our trust. Some controlling women won't ever be worth our emotional trust and some men won't be either. But there are some very defensive men and women who may be able to let go of controlling, given a change of experience and an awareness of their altered response to it."

"Well, I'll stick to animals for the rest of my days," stated Annie firmly. "They seem much more trustworthy than people to me."

"I know what you mean, Annie," sighed Jenny. "I don't think my gut is very reliable. After all, I have a steady track record of choosing the wrong men. It's me that I trust least of all, now, because my judgement appears to be absolutely useless when it comes to rotter spotting. The most I hope for these days, in terms of self esteem and companionship, is to get myself into a group of artists who will accept my presence among them. There's a new venture being advertised near me at the moment – an Artists' Cooperative – but the thought of applying to become a member and then being turned down is just unbearable. I don't think I'll ever pluck up enough courage to apply. Much safer to do my clay work on my own, in my little brick cellar! I'll stick to animals, too! I'm planning a series of paintings of my nephew's two goats when I get fed up with the clay work I'm doing of hens."

"Oh, are you sculpting hens at the moment?"

Annie sounded enthusiastic and as Jenny nodded, she suddenly rose to her feet. "Look, do come and see my work-station in the conservatory! I'm designing tapestry patterns based on Welsh country scenes, and the one I'm just starting is a farm yard. It took me a while to get a handle on the software but now I think I'm beginning to get the idea of it. Would you like to see what I'm doing?"

The invitation seemed to be addressed to Jenny in particular, and both women soon made their way out of the kitchen towards the French windows opening up onto the garden, chatting about the merits of computer software as they walked. Bianca and Alex remained sitting, but paused their conversation in order to allow the other the chance to join the conservatory party if she so desired. Neither made to leave, and Alex nodded towards Bianca with a smile.

"You were saying? About trusting your gut, and the benefit of the doubt?" she prompted, encouraging Bianca to continue.

"Oh yes! Well, it seems to me that none of our damaged men was ever going to be able to give women the benefit of the doubt, in the longer term. Maybe all these men that we were involved with were doing a sort of pre-emptive strike to ensure they took over the control when the relationship road got even ever so slightly bumpy.

"Something had happened – in their life experiences, in their basic personality, in their wiring, in their hormone distribution, in their upbringing, in their cultural environment, in any other factor combined with any or none of these – goodness knows! – to make them defend themselves against possible destructive control from intimate others. But perhaps their defence gradually became so armed with weaponry that in time, it couldn't be distinguished from attack.

"The men we are talking about are in the minority, don't you think, Alex? Just as the majority of women who tend their children with loving 'duty of care' use control only to protect the youngsters and, over time, do their utmost to allow their children to develop their own self confidence and independence, in the way best suited to each individual kid."

Alex nodded, wishing momentarily that she herself fell into this category of motherhood.

"So a woman who sidesteps intimacy in order to exert relentless control over her man is the damaged exception," continued Bianca. "You seem anxious, Alex, to make the point that some women might be able to establish such domination over their men without resorting to bullying or violence of any obvious sort, and that they may thus get away with it more easily. But actually, the two men both of you described to us last night – Nicky and Marcus, was it? – seem to have been able to do this, too. So do some damaged men make use of more 'feminine' manipulative techniques to establish their domination?"

"Yes, our men are skilled all right, especially – er – it's Ricky, actually, and Marcus, who were much more practised controllers than either Joe or Liam – lads, really – the ones Jenny and I married back in our early 20's. And, with the more mature duo, it could be very subtle mind-game stuff, indeed! I suppose that controlling men tend to start manipulating at a skill level which reflects how cleverly their first caregivers manipulated them. So perhaps male controllers who are brutal were themselves, as little ones, often beaten or whipped or controlled in some other very obviously damaging way. The raging, violent sort of partner probably won't, as a child, have experienced highly sophisticated tactics of control which make use of subtlety rather than brute force.

"In some cases, of course, the mums weren't the actual aggressors at all, but sometimes they simply did nothing to stop forceful aggression from another source, for a variety of reasons. It appears that the apparent failure to defend their dependent little one may be unconsciously bitterly resented by their child for ever after, however excusable this inaction may have been. Or maybe the mums deserted their kids or neglected them terribly or engulfed them completely.

"As far as I know, Jenny's Joe and Ricky both seem to have had good mums, but I think Joe had to spend a lot of time with his adoring grandma for some reason, when he was very small, and Jenny thinks that's what did for him. Can't have helped, either, that she describes Joe's father as a weak man; a dithering dreamer who acted the part of a distinguished doctor, and held court at the local pub as if he was a town celebrity.

"Ricky's Irish parents both seemed to have been good people.

His father was hugely admired and respected in Cork, and was one of the leading lights in the founding of the Cork Arts Festival. Jenny met him on one of her visits with Ricky, and she said he seemed a lovely man, with a deep affection for all three of his sons. His wife was dead by that time, remembered vividly by her family. Jenny got the impression that she had been regarded as great crack and a born entertainer. But I think Ricky said she wasn't a demonstrative woman at all, as far as her sons were concerned. There seems to have been some deep resentment between the brothers, and Ricky was the middle kid; something went wrong there somewhere, too. I think Ricky was his mum's favourite; second born but king pin until his little brother arrived who, in his turn, became the apple of his mother's eye. Their father got a job quite distant from home for a few years around about that time. So perhaps what happened was that young Ricky felt suddenly deprived of both parents' attention, and very jealous of this upstart baby, as the apparent cause of all this upheaval.

"As for my two Narcissists, Liam and Marcus, they had an amazing amount in common, as far as parental attitudes are concerned. Both mothers simply worshipped them, while both fathers, in different ways, tried unsuccessfully to compete with their only sons. Marcus's dad was very much dominated by his wife, who considered her husband to be a professional and social liability. Little Marcus, in contrast, could do no wrong! I think his dad alternated between trying to bond with his clever little son against the 'wimmin gang' – his wife and two daughters – and bitterly resenting how these three women idolised the boy of the family.

"And my first husband's dad was equally jealous of his only son's privileged place in the family spotlight, treasured by his mother and older sister. It's quite easy to see what went wrong there with both my beloved men. Those two conflicting messages of utter devotion and bitter resentment from mother and father must make a pretty toxic mixture. No wonder the kid grows up to blow hot and cold."

"So, in that case, they're just re-enacting what was done to them as children, by – um – a sort of clashing combination of attitudes, you think?" asked Bianca.

"More or less," nodded Alex. "I think all of us do that, really. We repeat what was done to us as very young kids or how we reacted to what we saw being done around us, unless we subsequently work out what formative stuff was happening in our childhood. If we're able to do that, we may then consciously decide either that we'll build on some element of our upbringing which provided a positive example, or that we'd rather do something else when our turn comes to be parents. We may, of course cherish some aspects of our parents' or grandparents' interpersonal dynamics, while rejecting others. But much more often, we are quite unaware of any of these considerations.

"When, as adults, deeply damaged sons or daughters first seek to form a new family type relationship, they can probably make a conscious effort to interact with sensitivity and intelligence. But I suspect that, in the case of people with severe attachment problems, the adult partnership gradually begins to take on the same sort of acidity as existed in their original family.

"That's all in their heads, of course. The present day relationship may be serenely alkaline in reality, but that healthiness won't be superimposed on the original version; instead, it'll work the other way round. And once that happens, the old damaging power systems are triggered off unconsciously, but this time, the one-time victim takes on the role of the oppressor, rather than the oppressed. If their parent was a punisher, a batterer or a deserter, they eventually find their own version of the same behaviour. Once they have started on this course, it appears there isn't much option for the oppressed person cast in the retrospective role of child victim. She has to get out.........."

Alex faltered to a pause, very conscious that she was on Bianca's territory here. Bianca nodded, acknowledging this fact, before taking up the theme.

"And yet we stay on, year after year, denying within ourselves that things are getting progressively worse, and always believing the relationship might change for the better. I don't think Andy was often physically punished or battered, but I think that family circumstances due to his mum's death gave him a terrible emotional battering, very early in his life. Maybe he was furious with her for dying, though he never acknowledged that to me. I never really thought about the long term impact of her death much, when I was still with him, I'm afraid. He never talked about his childhood, other than in the context of a beef about smokers. What I knew of it came mostly from his aunt, who was a lovely woman; we had many a good natter back in the early days of my marriage.

"I wish I'd tried to understand better what lay behind Andy's hitting out at me, and what a tsunami it would become for us, instead of concentrating on makeshift strategies to adapt to the situation somehow. It's so hard to recognise that things will tend to spiral downwards into deterioration. It's only once we begin to get more seriously bashed about that the need to get out becomes more glaringly obvious, I suppose, for our own physical survival. But *your* four men weren't using physical violence, were they? Did that make it hard for you to see any obvious reason to get out, even if you felt unhappy at times? Does it mean you both hung on in there until they walked out on you?"

"Absolutely right! How clever of you to see that, Bianca! Jenny and I were both abruptly deserted first time round. With the second whack of dysfunctional collusion, in my case, I just kept thinking I would be happy in our loving friendship if I could only keep Marcus happy. If I sensed he was discontent, somehow that must be my failure, never his. He had grown up as a 'special' child because he was the first born, the only son, and by far the most obviously intellectually gifted of the three siblings, and, incidentally, of most other children, too. His mother and younger sisters seemed to acknowledge his needs as paramount in the family. I think his father had never achieved any professional or social standing, much to his wife's exasperation, and his depressive bouts meant that he gradually began to slip into chronic failure, as seen through his family's eyes, anyway.

"Because of that, perhaps young Marcus got used to the idea that, in the face of his father's apparent shameful downfall, he himself represented the great hope of achievement for their little family. Perhaps he felt he could engineer a return to the high status days of his grandparents, who had, on both sides, stood out among their peers in terms of intellect and talent. (His paternal grandfather had read History at Oxford, and his mum's father had been a marine engineer.)

"I think all this meant that Marcus was always trying to live up to females' admiring expectations of him, but yet, I think he yearned to be secure in the male world too, accepted by his father and uncles, and allowed just to be an ordinary little boy. Instead, his uncles mocked him, claiming he was a sissy and calling him 'The Little Ponce'. And his father resented his glittering prizes throughout his school career, and the joy these gave his beleaguered mother. Maybe that's why, during the short time I had of knowing him, Marcus had a sort of cycle with me of pulling me into his personal life and then suddenly pushing me out again – blowing hot and cold.

"I guess he saw Love in his family as meaning inclusion for him but exclusion for his father, and he must have felt in conflict over that. Maybe he had to pay women back for what those family women had done to him: built him up like a king (pulled him forward) and thereby make him totally unacceptable to his displaced father in the process (getting him pushed back). The more his women folk applauded his constant triumphs, the more painfully Marcus must have felt cut off from the father who was becoming increasingly alienated from his family all the time.

"In the last year of his relationship with me, Marcus did little 'chucks' of me about once every two months – usually by an abrupt email – and then there would be a sustained silence over the airways; I never protested, of course. But after a few hours, days or weeks, he would suddenly email me again, the contents changed back to the delicious, lovey dovey stuff again, to my intense relief.

"If I asked him gently why he had just done one of these turn arounds, which I occasionally dared to do, he would say rather bleakly that he didn't know. I found him totally bewildering, and used to long to know if it was only me who felt that about him. But I could hardly ask his family about his capacity for personal consistency, could I! I knew there were people from his past and his present academic and professional worlds who very much disliked him, and even shunned him, but I presumed some of them might just be very envious of his acclaimed public reputation.

"So I carried on in our private world of tender intimacies, maintained for much of the time over the airways. We were good at daily romantic emails, both of us, though I suspect he often found mine rather too tedious to read much beyond the first sentence! There was an amazing ten or eleven weeks before the end when he did absolutely no dismissals at all, and I remember kidding myself that he had finally been 'loved out' of that neurotic cycle of Pull/Push behaviour. Actually, of course, he was just building up for the final chop!"

"But they don't know what they're doing, do they?" enquired Bianca. "They seem to me to be compelled to become controlling bullies, in some form or another. I eventually came to realise how Andy was building up the terror stakes bit by bit, but I don't think he had the remotest idea about what he was up to."

"No, I think that's right; they aren't consciously aware of the compulsion that's driving them to tighter and tighter control of the other person. Non-violent, 'gentlemen players' like Jenny's and mine may well have been tightly controlled as children, but I guess that the type of manipulative strategies used in the family would be far removed from any obvious bullying. It's much more often mind-games, such as the blowing hot and cold, which I experienced Marcus playing out on me.

"There are those reproachful, manipulative refrains in family dynamics which can undermine a young child's developing sense of Self by playing on his early vulnerability to guilt and shame. 'You've let us down badly by losing that egg and spoon race' or 'You break your mum's heart when you won't eat her roast potatoes' or 'Your poor little sister's got asthma because of those times you pinched her as a baby' – that sort of thing.

"Sometimes it's the opposite scenario in that the child is constantly shielded from any breathe of guilt or shame, as if he were a little god. 'If your teacher is telling you that you were wrong to spit at her, she'll have me to answer to!' The net result, at either extreme, is that the child can't learn to deal with his feelings on his own behalf.

"Caregivers who operate from either of these standpoints ('You never get it Right' or 'You can't get it Wrong') with their kids usually do so quite unconsciously and they are, God help 'em, doomed to pass on unprocessed family dysfunctions which they themselves probably experienced when they were children. Gentlemen players like Marcus and Ricky were, as kids, apparently able to develop a winning strategy of self protection. They became consummate players, hiding the Self which would, in a healthy environment, have been encouraged to adapt and learn from their little human errors or successes, in their own familiar environment.

"This concealment of their real Self keeps their emotional intelligence hopelessly arrested at toddler stage. The player version of the kid becomes more and more smoothly skilled at saying what the parent – or eventually, the chosen mate – wants to hear, and living up or down to what is required. These children have learnt to their cost that guilt and shame will never be managed alongside them in – er – the sort of loving steps which reflect a gentle combination of empathy and common sense. Because of this, they feel compelled to avoid any words or actions of theirs which could bring out the red Guilt or Shame Card against them, or topple them from their established perch.

"When this same child seeks to create a family type relationship as an adult, he will know all the tricks of the trade, as far as delight and charm are concerned. He will often choose a partner who seems to have some natural flair in areas he feels himself to be lacking. This makes the pressure of maintaining his imposing false front much less exhausting for him because he can assimilate his partner's genuine gifts, along with the ones he is demonstrating on his own behalf, making himself feel more rounded.

"But once again, things will go wrong if he begins to invest in a deeper two way relationship with such a partner. The partner intimacy may not be anything like the subversive controlling of his childhood, and, to start with, might bring out his most skilful role play relevant to this new, healthy relationship's requirements, while that tucked away toddler Self will be held in check, as far as he can manage it. He may be required to play the perfect devoted husband, father and family man/soul mate which he can often sustain successfully for decades!"

"Andy certainly held all that together for our first ten years," remarked Bianca, sighing as she rested her head on one hand.

"As time goes on, however, holding these two parts of himself separate becomes more and more difficult for him," continued Alex.

"Kids grow up, his own parents die, careers paths alter, age adds to tums and chins and takes away from scalp covering. He cannot process the feelings attached to these inevitable challenges in life because he has never learnt how to work through and come to terms with disappointment and loss. His role playing consistency begins to crack. As this happens, his destructive impulses from the repressed toddler Self begin to seep out, little by little.

"His partner may become more and more puzzled and confused by his increasingly un-integrated ways of relating. He may peer at her eyelashes unexpectedly and make a childlike comment such as, 'A few of them are bunched together with a blobby black dot.'

This sort of observation may directly follow a delicately worded critique of her earlier telephone conversation with a colleague, or a casual comment about his need to get his car serviced. It appears to the listener to be pretty disjointed stuff.

"Sometimes his spoken sentences themselves may seem to lack structural coherence. This peculiarity is labelled 'Word salad' in some analytical circles, and it means that various different ingredients seem to be chucked into the mixture in a rather random way, muddling the flavour of what is being said. It's an interesting label, isn't it? This mixing happens particularly when the player is required to comment on anything personal, where a genuine emotional response seems relevant. His partner may subsequently discover that the seepage goes far beyond incongruous comments or phrasing. He may turn out to have been increasingly involved in internet porn, or 'swinging' or 'cottaging' or some other secret activity which allows that long suppressed side of himself, that gleeful, naughty childish rebellion, as it were, full rein."

"I seem to remember Charles Dickens having a sort of secret life, in a biography I read about him," commented Bianca, finger outstretched. "What you're saying reminds me of him needing another world – I think he had a young mistress in the theatre – where he could duck out of playing the high profile, admired Man of Letters. So maybe it's common for damaged controllers to feel straddled between two worlds, and to become split somehow between two dimensions as a result? And what about Edward VIII? He did the same with Wallis Simpson, didn't he? He could hardly have chosen a woman more likely to cause a split between his private desires and his public role.

"The realms of royalty must provide a fertile breeding ground for damaged personality, mustn't it? All that public recognition, yet lots of private angst and huge parental expectation and psychological deprivation."

"Yes, indeed!" Alex agreed, with alacrity. "There may well be a disproportionate number of Narcissists among royalty, the priesthood and the acting profession, I would have thought. And we apparently live in a 'Celebrity Culture' where being narcissistic is pretty acceptable in society; indeed, it is often positively encouraged and rewarded. But people with Narcissistic Personality Disorder rarely sound happy, however celebrated they are. Some of the things Peter Sellers said about feeling empty if he wasn't performing are very poignant, and make it sound as if he actually knew that a grounded sense of Self was tragically far beyond his reach.

"They say that Marilyn Monroe and Princess Diana might both have suffered from an inability to engage in close personal relationships without an obsessive terror of abandonment. Some experts claim that emotional flooding like that is the flipside of Narcissistic Personality Disorder, with an equally odd label of 'Borderline'. The conditions can both be classified as disorders of the Self. The early deaths of both Diana and Marilyn Monroe suggest that one way or another, they didn't take enough precautions about their own lives, physically or emotionally, and perhaps that's because, at root, they felt betrayed by some of the adults they had loved as very young children.

"Diana wasn't wearing her safety belt when she was killed, d'you remember? At some buried level of awareness, did she not think her own safety worth preserving? Both those women were caught between a public image of adorable, enchanting beauty and a private turmoil of insecurity and self destruction. Again, we're up against a huge split in how they were seen and how they actually felt inside."

Bianca took up this theme fervently.

"Well, in his less glittering environment, my Andy also got himself caught between two extremes; the outdoor working life of a man supporting his family as best he can, and a large business enterprise where corporate success overtook him, somehow. It seemed like he couldn't find a way to integrate those two worlds without seeking somehow to destroy one of them, and it was the ordinary working life which had to go. He seemed to have to split our family into all good or all bad, too; there was no middle ground for him.

"At first, we looked as if we could be the ideal little set up in his mind, but once Stephen got into just that little bit of trouble, it seemed like it triggered off a need in Andy to destroy the whole fabric of our lives as a family, bit by bit. It's literally as if he was disintegrating. He couldn't bring together the peaks and troughs which seem to me to be an inevitable part of family life, as years go by. You could say that disappointment and loss somehow blew his circuitry."

"That idea of 'splitting' is a pretty vital factor in all this," agreed Alex, lighting on Bianca's words with intense interest. "I must say, I've found it a hard one to get to grips with. It can work at the most mundane of levels, in the subtlest of ways, and can easily be misconstrued. I remember I used to be very puzzled when I was parting from Marcus after another lovely morning together, and we would hug each other and seem to share a sadness about saying farewell. He might then suddenly remark, 'Those socks you're wearing – they look totally naff, you know.' To be fair, Bianca, they probably did! I'm careless about socks and even shoes, because I think they won't show; ordinary and boring will do!

"But for him to make an unexpected remark like that in the context of tender farewells seemed to me – well – odd. D'you know what I mean? Eventually, I decided that it must be that he didn't like parting from me, and this was his indirect way of expressing his pain.

"Now I see that it was probably quite different! All morning he would have been suppressing any urge to 'side swipe' with a 'nah nah' type criticism because his chosen role with me was that of gently romantic literary lover, but he couldn't quite last out three hours before the toddler Self had to emerge for a quick spontaneous jab. He had been struggling to suppress the impulsive jabber under his guise of eloquent romantic, but they are difficult extremes to hold apart for long. He didn't seem able to find a position in the middle but instead, sought to maintain the split which put him under enormous pressure at times.

"When I was first his targeted woman, I was put on a pedestal by him and repeatedly credited with making him feel a joyful, liberated person. During that pedestal and take-over phase, the woman – me, Jenny, whoever – may feel worshipped and appreciated as never before. She may even feel that having the best of her characteristics merging with his is the ultimate loving act between two human beings, exceeding even the transient bliss of sexual connection. Some survivors say that it's like living in paradise when you are fused with a partner in this all-embracing way.

"Maybe it has some sort of echo back to the time when you were incorporated within the abundant supplies of the womb? There is a theory that we are all constantly seeking to regain that feeling! Anyway, the state is like being high on the most powerful of drugs, and equally addictive.

"I expect it happens because the predator is often solely, relentlessly, obsessively targeting this new supplier. He has none of the small distractions and breaks in concentration that 'normal' people may be diverted by, even when they also are beginning to fall for a new person in their lives.

"It is very rare for us ever to be in the full beam of another person's attention in that sort of way, and we may well bask in the glare of it, instead of being able to identify it as a kind of soul stalking. That was a big factor in my addiction to Marcus; he initially seemed somehow utterly fascinated by even the tiniest aspect of me. I remember that right from the start of our relationship, he would sometimes suddenly peer at me closely and then lean forward with a finger to flick away a tiny speck of something ('sleep', perhaps?) from the inner corner of my eye. I think I may have felt a slight surprise when he did that, but I didn't really register it.

"In retrospect, it seems a startling invasion of space between two adults who are only just getting to know one another, but I think I had already somehow allowed a strange merging of our individual identities to take place. And I came to feel only half alive without him, though this effect lessened if we were separated for quite a while because of summer holidays or something like that. It never occurred to me that actually, I was chronically weakened by being with him, and that I grew stronger in myself out of his company, especially during a fortnight's holiday abroad with Dan.

"Um – where was I? Oh yes – addiction! The trouble is, the more of her characteristics he appropriates, the less the player actually comes to value *her* because there is no need at all for him to see her as separate from him. He adopts the best of her ways and she begins to feel impoverished. He gradually comes to have little use for what is only the husk of her. Eventually, she is discarded and he starts – or restarts – the whole process again with someone else. She is left with the worst agonies of PTSS and drug-withdrawal, combined in a catastrophic psychological mix which doesn't get treated effectively because it is rarely correctly diagnosed.

"It may appear to be deliberate manipulation, but I really believe the effect of his fragmented Self on the woman is not actually planned out by this sort of player, as you've already pointed out, Bianca. He may be operating in a smooth, orderly way on other levels, but his feeling/memory/reflective capacities are deeply impaired. This means that his internal emotional life is chaotic, despite his finely honed talent for disguising this from others.

"Actually, there is a commonality in predators, however much their individual personalities and environments may differ. They will always have to resort to the use of overt or covert power and control in their personal relationships. This is because personal relationships, at the deepest level, are intensely threatening to them, and players will be reduced, in time, to the frequent use of primitive defences such as splitting, for self protection from perceived attack. It is these very defences which stultify them, arresting their psychological development.

"Theirs is the tragedy, in the end, because the victim may be able to become a survivor, but predators are much less likely ever to be able to release themselves from the overbearing weight of their own weaponry. It's strange and ironic to reflect that in suppressing their capacity to feel pain, players inadvertently destroy the essence of their humanity and any chance of moving alongside loved ones and other like-minded people in a real experience of connection and development. Somewhere inside himself, the predator senses this mutilation and he constantly seeks to escape the horror and emptiness of it, but as it is coming from inside him, there is nowhere he can run to.

"The best a player like Marcus can achieve, in terms of feeling, is to project a response of his own onto someone else, and try to release himself a little in the observation of the other's reactive feelings. That way, at least he gets to experience the odd moment of emotional intensity by proxy. A good example of that is when Marcus once showed me a bit of his daughter's wedding DVD. He focused on his wife's facial expression as she listened to apparently moving words delivered by the best man at the wedding speeches section. Marcus seemed to get some sort of buzz by watching how Tessa's face was registering emotion and he paused the clip to repeat it, urging me more than once to observe that she was close to tears but fighting them back. Weird stuff, really.

"Sorry, I'm banging on again. It's the survival of the victim which is the essential thing, not the complexities of the dysfunctional person's condition, but I'm always getting sidetracked by intriguing anomalies like that! Where was I? Er – for the targeted person, the switching from feeling warmly cocooned in a golden love bubble to being stripped of one's very identity is, at first hint, destabilising and eventually – when the ice takes its fiercest, final grip – devastating. But that sense of emptiness is probably an unconscious picking up of the controller's own inner turmoil, projected onto her. There is nothing personal in his annihilation of the other. He simply has no further use for her. It's very hard to get your head round it all."

"So what about gay relationships?" mused Bianca. "Can a man gain this sort of subtly abusive power over a male partner, or a female over another woman? Would the fact that they're the same gender affect the dynamic you're describing?"

"I really don't know much about this first hand, or through friends. I know a little about it through counseling but I haven't read it up or anything. In training, we were told about a gay relationship where one woman client was very much the controller and initially unwilling to respect the rights of the appeasing other, but their issues seemed to be related to their contrasting responses to their dominating mothers. Once that was examined, the problems apparently resolved quite quickly, and the relationship moved forward in renewed mutual understanding. So I don't think relationship dysfunction could have been the issue there.

"I haven't yet come across male gay couples in my counseling. Maybe the gender thing applies here, in that many men seem particularly reluctant to analyse their responses in relationships, so a male couple might be doubly unwilling to do so – I really don't know. I do remember one case I read about where a man came for counselling on his own, saying he was determined to leave his wife of many years, but he didn't know why. He seemed absolutely tortured, and described his wife as a lovely woman who was hugely upset to learn he was planning to leave her and their almost adult children.

"He acknowledged that he might well be making the wrong decision but that he didn't care; he just had to do something. He said he felt like he was being sucked down through a dark void and was losing control of his own responses. When I read that, I thought that maybe I recognised that description, and I wondered if there could be some dysfunction in another person connected with him which was damaging him at close quarters. It turned out, later in the account, that his older brother had been a pathological controller over him all his young life. The younger man had escaped from this control by going into the services at seventeen but events had occurred within the last ten years which had brought his brother very much back into the frame.

"Well, it transpired that the older brother held a fearsome indirect control over the younger one still, and that this younger brother was actually going into 'bewilderment spinning' – the same feeling that Jenny and I know so well. But as this guy had never worked out what his older brother's dysfunction had originally done to his own mental health, he'd never considered that there could be any collateral damage which would be reawakened with any further brotherly contact.

"So he didn't recognise toxic aftermath or PTSS or whatever you like to call it, and just thought it must be his marriage; it was the only explanation he could come up with. So there you have male on male controlling, with the victim mistakenly identifying his wife as the threat, against all his own instincts and the plain evidence to the contrary. Interesting, don't you think?"

"I suppose in that case, it's a man just expecting to be somewhat dominated by a woman, as usual. So if he actually begins to register feeling unaccountably bewildered and empty, he jumps to the conclusion that she must somehow be smothering him completely, and he needs to get out."

Bianca paused and then continued to explore the theme, looking across at Alex with bright-eyed interest.

"I wonder if that same conclusion lies behind some young men going along the gay route where they aren't actually gay by nature, if you know what I mean. Maybe some men are aware of rather too intense a bond with their mothers and subconsciously protect themselves by subsequently seeking intimacy exclusively with other men?

"They might see it as a way of avoiding too tight a control being held over them. Do you think there may be even more gay men who choose to lead their romantic lives with men, now that many of the young women surrounding them seem more feisty about their own lives and careers, and have much more choice than their mothers and grandmothers in the previous generations?"

"Pretty sad, though, isn't it?" replied Alex. "It seems rather gloomy to me, if the long term survival of our genes through successful reproduction depends to some extent on the female's mind set of basic submission to chance or to the male's control! For centuries, the power balance, in most of Western society at least, has been that way round, especially with women having no reliable means of contraception available. That has meant that sexually active women were producing babies – and sometimes dying in the process – all the time.

"Now that science and society have combined to make having a child more of a choice for women, rather than an obligation, it could be that it's men who hold back from the whole heterosexual bonding bit. Equality of the power balance, whether in domestic or professional arenas, must be pretty scary for men, especially if it's breaking the pattern of generations."

Alex paused, feeling uncomfortable with how theoretically she was speaking. Her personal experience of family life seemed a possible antidote to generalities, and she quickly harnessed it.

"I was quite lucky, actually! Although my dad was powerful and rather bad tempered, my mum managed him very skilfully, quietly achieving her own agenda in her own time, and understanding that his temper outbursts were temporary blips which would soon be followed by an apology. As a couple, they were generally very affectionate and devoted to one another, too. Somehow the power balance evened itself out between them rather well. I think that's why I'm pretty optimistic about romantic relationships, even though I've made terrible choices twice over."

"And do you think both of you are safe now, from Marcus and Ricky?" enquired Bianca gently. "I gather each of them was the one to terminate the relationship, but you say that men like them don't base their actions on their inner feelings in any reflective way. Doesn't that mean they might pop back into your lives at some point in the future, expecting to pick up where they left off?

"After all, they haven't been violent or stolen your credit cards or set fire to your garden fence! They may not register causing any serious hurt or harm because they weren't husbands deserting their wives and they hadn't made any formal commitment. They might circle round for another go, if circumstances made that expedient for them, mightn't they? What would either of you do then?"

"Oh, I'm sure we would see them," replied Alex swiftly. "My long suffering husband would hate it, but he wouldn't prevent me. I've already told him that I would want to meet with Marcus again at least once, if he ever asked me to. I've said I would need to do that, finally to stop obsessing about it, constantly trying to make sense of it.

"Believe it or not, there's still a tiny part of me which maintains the hope that perhaps Marcus and I could be true friends to one another! I loathe losing a deep friendship, you see; it horrifies me. I think I'll only ever wipe that hope out as a possibility if I get another chance to try for it. Daft, isn't it? Dan says it'll only do my head in all over again, but I really believe that Jenny and I are too vigilant about our own well-being to put our sanity at risk once more. I can't see Marcus coming back, though; I'm of no further use to him. But Ricky might return to Jenny, I think, if things go wrong with the Spanish lady.

"In the stuff I've read, it says just what you're suggesting, Bianca. Apparently, these garden variety pretenders often do circle round for one or more courtship assault on a previous target. Maybe they want to see if they can still regain control, even though they've previously dropped and shattered the target as useful supply. Heady stuff, very empowering and confirming for them, if they can win control all over again! Perhaps they've just lost an alternative possibility for encroachment, and find themselves reduced to recycling a provider they abandoned earlier. It's certainly a lovely opportunity for them to play Freezing Cold to being Passionately Hot again, and to watch the erstwhile supplier's dazed response; delight on the one hand, wounded wariness on the other. Apparently, it often happens. The supplier believes that this time, things will be different. Maybe they are, for a while."

"And a rejected woman who loves her man is likely to see virtue in forgiveness, isn't she?" observed Bianca. "Perhaps she'll begin to take on all the blame for the break up in the first place. She might even take the blame repeatedly, determined to maintain the eternal hope of making it work."

"Yes, you're absolutely right! I know of one woman, a cousin of Jenny's actually, who was dumped by her Narcissist husband after nearly thirty years of marriage. She was heart scalded. He went off travelling and created a new identity for himself as a palaeontologist somewhere in South Africa for a while, with no such professional expertise whatsoever! He had left Evelyn to rebuild her life, slowly and painfully, with help from very good friends such as Jenny. Evelyn eventually got stronger and surer of her capacity to flourish on her own, and was beginning to recover.

"Meanwhile, things weren't going at all well any more for the adventurer. After several years, he returned to Hampshire in a camper van, and slept in it, in the railway car park nearest his former marital home, for at least a year. Gradually, he began to ingratiate his way back into Evelyn's life, doing odd jobs, D.I.Y., cutting the lawn, you know. And slowly, slowly, the whole question of where he was based became fudged as he began to encroach on what used to be their shared home.

"Now it's about a dozen years later, and he's back in place, ruling the roost, as if he was never away. He has never referred to why he left or why he returned; it's a closed subject. And she's the contented little woman, serving his needs, secure in having her man back. They've reinvented themselves as a happy couple, enjoying their retirement. He's prepared to play the role required of cosy husband, for the sake of regaining a comfortable life. And his wife has forgotten what it was like to open the window and feel the fresh breeze on her face."

"And is that really so bad a compromise?" asked Bianca, after a pause. "If he's too old to go a wandering again, maybe he can keep up the role for the rest of his days. And if that's how she wants him to be, isn't that......"

But the reflection was interrupted here by the return of the others, Annie moving swiftly up to her friend to place a hand on her shoulder.

"Before they set off, could Jenny and Alex pop into your house and see some of your exhibition work? I've been telling Jenny about it and she'd love a glimpse, wouldn't you, Jenny?"

"Oh yes! It sounds amazing! It's quilting, but not as you and I know it," Jenny explained, for Alex's benefit.

"Well, of course you can, if you'd really like to, replied Bianca. "It's just a lot of stitching, you know. But have you got time? You were hoping to set off shortly, weren't you?"

"Oh, as long as we're on the road within the next hour, we'll be fine," replied Jenny, adding, "Would that really be okay, Bianca? If we settle up here, pack up, and call in then? But what about your husband? Won't we be intruding?"

"He's in his work den already; he won't mind a bit. He might even come down. He has become pretty adept at explaining the history of quilting himself, since I took it up. What about you, Annie? You've seen it all dozens of times...."

"Oh no; I want to come as well!"

"Fine! I'll be off then, and see you all shortly."

Bianca rose to her feet somewhat stiffly, keeping her back in an upright position as she moved. Then she gave them all a wide grin and turned to leave the room.

Jenny and Alex were soon at Annie's threshold, car packed up, bill paid, and agreeing with Annie that she would walk the few steps down the hill to Bianca's house while Jenny and Alex drove the car down into Bianca's driveway, poised in position for their subsequent departure. They had barely stepped out of the car again when Bianca was alongside them, ushering them inside her house and turning back to welcome Annie in as well.

It was a square, modern house, in stark contrast to Annie's, somewhat dark inside at first but leading into huge amounts of space and a view onto woodland at the back, through a large expanse of floor to ceiling window. There was a predominance of dark wood in the living room, as if there was not much difference between the outside and inside world. The room was uncluttered and there was little sign of it being used for daily domesticity. In the centre of this sizeable interior was a wide coffee table with two low stools pushed alongside it to create an even larger surface. And draped carefully over it was a huge expanse of quilt, mainly blue in colour. Another one of similar size had been positioned over the brown leather three piece suite, some distance away in the corner.

"I just pulled out two," said Bianca, nodding towards her work. "If you want to see any more, it's easy to show them to you, but it's a bit of a fiddle getting them back in their drawers again."

She nodded towards a set of huge built-in cupboards with layer upon layer of long, narrow drawers. These looked to Alex to be custom made for holding their contents. Jenny was already standing over the blue quilt, asking and gaining permission to examine it through a momentary exchange of head gestures between herself and Bianca, before starting her closer inspection. She took in the complexity of the central hexagonal design, the beauty of the blended shades of blue, the variety of materials used and the exquisite combination of art and craft and precision which the quilt displayed. There was a pause.

"This is wonderful!" she exclaimed, turning back to Bianca. "I've never seen quilting like this!"

Annie looked pleased with herself for having provided this opportunity. She nodded, smiling across at Bianca and declaring,

"Knocks spots off my little quilted cushions!"

Alex had moved forward to survey the other end of the blue quilt. She had no experience of decorative sewing, unlike the other three, but the artistry of the work was immediately obvious.

"This must have taken you years to make, didn't it?" she breathed, overawed by the quilt's vastness and yet its meticulous attention to detail. Every single one of its many hexagons had hand-stitched embroidery embellishing its edges and centre.

"Well, I don't tend to make such heavy pieces now, because of my back trouble. That one I did about eight years ago now, I think. It was one of my first, and in those days, I was much slower at it. I don't work at them every day, of course. But I'd guess, adding it all up, it took about a year to complete. I wasn't totally satisfied with it, but it certainly got me hooked on the craft. I had no idea before I started how much I'd get drawn into it all. Derek teases me that one day I'll find my tights firmly stitched up within a piece of work, with my legs still encased inside!"

"Come and look at this one; this was her second!" announced Annie, and the women followed her towards the gold and scarlet quilt on the sofa. "Bianca's work has been exhibited in the Quilt Museum at York. And she's regional coordinator for Wales."

"Not the whole of Wales," laughed Bianca. "I only run one region – Mid and South."

"Is there a national organisation of quilt makers, then?" enquired Alex, gazing at the exquisite blends of red and amber of the indicated spread.

"Oh yes! It's called the Quilters' Guild. The membership is divided into eighteen regions all over the United Kingdom, but we have an international section as well. We have all sorts of events, activities and exhibitions going on throughout the regions. It's surprising how many things you can get involved in, if you're keen enough on quilting!"

"And how many members do you have, roughly? Jenny enquired.

"Oh, about seven thousand, I think," replied Bianca.

"Seven thousand?" Alex repeated, taken aback that a craft which she knew virtually nothing about should attract such a large membership.

"Yes! Well, it was founded thirty years ago. So its membership has had plenty of time to develop over that time, and it has achieved quite a lot, really, in terms of education about the history of quilting in Great Britain. For example, we've built up a collection of hundreds of pieces of quilting, dating from this year back to the early eighteenth century."

"So it's not just bedspreads, then?"

"Oh no! Our museum in York displays all sorts of pieces: clothing, appliqué hangings, coverlets, quilting tools, domestic items, fabrics, documents, patterns and photos. There's lots there for researchers, if they want to find out things at that sort of level. We often get visitors from the States and Canada, looking into the history of decorative folk art. Quilting really took off in the New World, of course, back in the eighteenth and nineteenth centuries. People sometimes assume that the Guild just focuses on impoverished English peasant women desperately stitching together material scraps for bed coverings, but it has a much wider remit than that."

"Show them some of your other stuff!" urged Annie, and soon Alex and Jenny were standing in front of the long wooden drawers and watching as piece after piece was edged gently out into full view. There were small cot covers, single bed quilts, quilted pictures and hangings of every shape and size and design. The range of fabrics, colours, and illustrative designs was surprisingly varied. Some pieces had a whimsical quality, while others had an ornate formality, with their traditional border designs and elaborate symbols. The radiance of their colours and the rich substance of their materials combined to illuminate the room, and the inner and outer space of the four women was soon sprinkled with images of swans and fish and rippling rivers and oceans with rolling breakers and radial beamed sunsets and starry moonscapes and undulating hills and countless other timeless images of grace and beauty.

As Alex tried to absorb the extent of Bianca's works of art, she glanced across at Jenny, and there was a brief exchange of raised eyebrows between them. Both women were aware of their limitations in response, since it was difficult to keep expressing admiration without simply repeating their appreciative exclamations. Jenny began to ask about particular techniques used in this piece or that, knowledgeable about some aspects of the craft already, but Alex had no such vocabulary available.

Her mind was already moving beyond what she could see in front of her to an indistinct image of the country's quilters, past and present, searching out their bits of fabrics and threads, and assembling them before starting work on a particular item. She imagined this confederation of women, scattered gradually throughout Britain and far beyond those shores, working individually, yet each seeking to piece together their various textile scraps into an integrated whole.

Sometimes they might be doing so for diversion, sometimes to earn some extra money, sometimes out of desperate poverty, or perhaps, like Bianca here, for the chance to express her creativity in an impressive range of colour coordinated fabrics and techniques. Alex was startled to realise that this was the first time she had ever had any concept of this particular shared activity, involving so many women over several centuries.

She was aware of the slight internal dizziness which she had come to recognise heralded a new connection within her somewhat unsatisfactory brain. Sometimes, the faint buzzing was the predominant experience and the realisation came much later, but on this occasion, it was easy to reach for enlightenment instantaneously. After all, the last fifteen hours in this particular location had been lived by both herself and Jenny at a somewhat heightened level of awareness, in any case. Their Well Head quest had appeared to reach its denouement the evening before, when they had registered that their targeted candidate for rescue, Annie, had already been taken tenderly under Bianca's protective wing. To add to the twist in the tale, the combined experience of the other two women had served to broaden their own perspectives about tactics used by a type of controller whom, despite their search for understanding, they had never seriously considered.

And now, here Alex was, faced with the outward and physical sign of an inward and spiritual truth: that we stitch together the fabric of our experiences best with the support of others who widen our frame of reference, and share our need to create something greater than the sum of the parts. This is what human beings do; they are sociable animals.

She was still somewhat dazed from this reflection as Jenny began to make departing noises. Bianca and Annie were both responding with warm wishes for the success of their research, and also for their safe return to Hampshire. Alex could, of course, join in these exchanges and did so, but she felt somehow slightly distanced from the others. She could hear from Jenny's tone that she was preparing for driving and navigating mode, and the other two women were perhaps already beginning to step back towards their normal Sunday routines. She moved into the dark corridor and turned, along with Jenny, to hug both their hostesses with reciprocated warmth.

As Jenny turned back to step through the opened front door, she paused, her eye caught by a small, narrow wall hanging just inside the threshold. It was an appliqué image of a stylized bird, wings outstretched, beak turned to one side. Even in the darkness of this interior space, the silver threads which embellished its wings glistened faintly. There was no need to ask if Bianca had created it, since it was evidently characteristic of her art.

"Oh, I like that one!" commented Jenny promptly, indicating the wall hanging above her as she passed it.

Bianca nodded with a smile and Annie moved alongside her, head resting briefly against her friend's shoulder.

"I knew you'd both love her work," she affirmed. "I'm so proud of my genius neighbour!"

"Ya daft dodo!" commented Bianca, shrugging slightly as if in denial of this praise, and thereby dislodging Annie's head. The friends remained side by side to watch as Jenny and Alex stepped into the car. As the engine started and Jenny steered their way gingerly out through the open gate, the two neighbours continued to wave, and their visitors returned the gesture enthusiastically until the intervening hedge blocked their view of the house. They were soon at the base of the slope and taking the first of many turns in the network of lanes which would eventually take them back to the main road.

"Okay?" said Jenny, with a brief glance across at Alex.

"Ready to roll!" replied Alex with a grin, and they set off on the long journey home.

EPILOGUE ONE

NEARLY TWO YEARS LATER

Alex's final walk with Marcus Spring 2008

Alex could feel his coldness as soon as Marcus waved at her, Beano on a lead at his side. His appearance charmed her as it always did: the immaculate and perfectly coordinated outdoor gear, the extra poised stance of a man of average height, the glow about his face, the fresh radiance of childhood about him somehow. And yet she felt chilled as she approached him. She wondered momentarily whether that coldness was coming from inside her and had nothing to do with him at all, but as she drew closer to him, she could see how his pose was rigid and wary, his smile too brief, his chin tilted slightly upward.

Her heart sank as she knew whatever she said or did now was futile; his defence against her would be impenetrable. It did mean, however, that she had nothing to lose. This afternoon's meeting was an inexplicable charade of his choosing, but she might as well use it to say what she felt, regardless of his response, because she knew she was nothing to him now.

She sank down to his side, greeting Beano warmly, and the little terrier snuffled sweetly against her, pushing his front paws onto her knees. It was a relief to feel this brief, affectionate connection before straightening up to stand eye to eye with his owner.

"He's very pleased to see you," commented Marcus, jerking the lead slightly.

"And I'm very pleased to see him, and his lovely master."

They kissed quickly once, cheek to cheek. She hesitated,

tempted to turn back towards her car straight away. A shaft of ice seemed to have pierced her stomach. She glanced across at him as he turned his back on her to start walking up the path. After a few paces, he paused and glanced back towards her, his eyebrows raised, mouth tight. She hastened towards him and they set off, Beano snuffling enthusiastically at the wooded side of the bridle path ahead of them. The early April colouring was muted; everything around them seemed to be a brownish grey or a sort of washed-out white, and there was no discernable scent of the countryside.

Alex felt as if she was walking in a vanished landscape. Or was it, she wondered, more like the Valley of the Shadow of Death? Her mind ran over the words of the 23rd Psalm. She couldn't feel any comfort from Marcus's rod or staff, despite the fact that he had it with him, as always, for protection against angry horses or bullocks. Nor could she claim that she feared no evil because in fact she felt in considerable psychological danger.

How had Scott Peck defined 'evil'? she asked herself, yet again, stumbling her way through a series of stony potholes in the mud. It was something about 'non love' being the emotional laziness of a fearful person whereas 'anti love' was evil; a deliberate exercising of power over another by overt or covert coercion. She felt she might actually be shaking, somehow destabilised by her mounting awareness of this 'anti love', but she tried to reason herself out of her agitation. Marcus had *asked* to meet her this afternoon, they had done this same walk in harmony many times before, Beano needed the exercise, his owner seemed disengaged and remote, rather than coercive or manipulating.

She was being ridiculous. She reached out to touch Marcus's fingers briefly. He had his stick in one hand and Beano's lead in the other, making it awkward for them to hold hands. He glanced at her sideways and smiled.

"Beano can't believe his luck," he commented lightly. "I've been very remiss about taking him for walks over the last few days; I just couldn't fit it in at all. Your master's useless, isn't he, Old Boy?"

"I think you've done brilliantly! You say you've got all the decoration done, and the shelving is nearly finished. It's amazing how you've achieved it all so quickly."

"Well, once I decide to do something, I don't hang around. It was always obvious what the top priority was – the safe and efficient shelving of all my books and manuscripts in the best possible conditions available for a unique private library. I know the right people to employ, of course, and I can manage a work-force without any hitches occurring. I just eliminate almost everything else from my agenda. I can cut off just like that, whatever else might be going on. It's very helpful, really, since it leaves no time for agonising or reconsidering."

Alex lit on this shard of self analysis inwardly, but paused before commenting tentatively,

"Might it be that you're wary of reconsidering, then? Sometimes we rush things through in order to trap ourselves into going with that decision......."

"Not in the least! I certainly didn't rush the decision about finding the right place. I read through at least three hundred property descriptions meticulously and was absolutely open-minded about where my base should be, other than within a fifteen mile radius of the cathedral, in any direction. That's hardly slapdash, you know. I've worked extremely hard to find somewhere which came as close as possible to my ideal, within the price range."

He seemed irritated, although his tone was even. She felt reprimanded and tried switching the subject.

"And Tessa? Does she seem okay about her new flat?"

"Oh yes! She loves it. It's a beautiful place. But of course she isn't able to have ol' Beano there. So that was another requirement I had to cope with. The place I needed to find had to be dog-friendly, since I am, perforce, in sole custody of the mastiff. There's no garden for him at The Courtyard, but it's only a one minute walk to the woods where he has acres to explore. The neighbours seem delightful, and they are very pro dogs, as far as I can see. On my second morning there, last Tuesday, a very elegant matron was walking past me as I was getting out of the car without Old Bean there. She greeted me by saying, 'Oh yes! I'd heard you were moving in – how nice. And is it a Yorkshire or a Staffordshire?' No interest in me at all! Bush telegraph stuff, I suppose. It's all very 'Horse and Hound'."

It was hard for Alex to find a response to this. She remembered how often he had mocked such people in the past, and yet now he was clearly determined to be embraced in their world.

"What about your statue?" she enquired eventually.

"Well, there's a corner of shrubbery to the side of my end wall, alongside the gates. There's room for my Saint Francis just there, to welcome in all visitors. I've asked four of the other seven Courtyard residents whether they would object and it's quite the contrary; they seem delighted. I'll wait until the other three sets of residents are around and I've consulted them before I set it up, though. It's an impressive way to introduce myself, actually, asking their permission to put up a beautiful and very valuable work of art to enhance their own environment. I think it might lead to an order or two for Harry Wagner because people are sure to ask me about the sculptor, and there's certainly no shortage of cash in the area, despite the fact that his prices are going up exponentially, in line with his reputation."

"But I suppose you wouldn't want anyone buying another Saint Francis, would you? Is he a one-off?"

"Well, no. There are six of them now, but I was the original commissioner. Harry and I subsequently agreed that he could cast five more if he dropped the price he initially proposed to charge me, to compensate. He was very decent about it all and most efficient; ex-army type, you know. I'll ask him to my housewarming do. He has become a friend now; you'd love him."

Alex noted that a party was planned and that she was evidently not to be included as a guest. She smiled wryly to herself. She had been right to think she was being phased out. Presumably the New Woman would not want her there either. There was a brief silence.

"Shall we take the woods route?" he asked, waving his stick towards the left. She nodded, and Beano approached his master to be let off the lead, tail wagging. He knew his doggy route well up through this path and, once off the lead, launched himself with gusto towards his first joyful sniffing area.

Now that Marcus was dog free, Alex moved a little closer beside him, but it was difficult to take the opportunity to speak of heart matters. She had little to lose, though, she reminded herself, since more superficial topics seemed to represent a mine field in any case. They walked in silence for a few moments. Her mind was running over the painful conclusions she had come to as to his real motives for asking to meet up again, towards the end of last year. It would be wonderful to be mistaken, but she feared she was not. She had guessed that she might serve as a useful weapon against any reproaches he might be subjected to from Tessa. The fact that his rejected romantic lover of three years ago would welcome him back as a beloved friend would surely be useful to him, serving as a model for how his wife should be expected to take their marriage breakdown.

It would probably be extremely painful for Tessa to be told that he had resumed his friendship with Alex, immediately the agreed separation had set him free to do so, and that she herself had jumped at the chance of their reunion. Alex suspected Marcus wanted to inflict that particular hurt on Tessa since the proposal of a six month trial separation had, according to him, first been reluctantly suggested by Tessa herself. 'Put up to it by that feminist therapist she has ensconced herself with!' was how he had phrased it contemptuously to Alex.

She also guessed that his New Woman, whatever her name was, had been lined up in the wings well before he had agreed to negotiate with Tessa for October's temporary parting of the ways. From the morning after the appointed date, it seemed that Marcus had dropped any preconceived notion that the separation was temporary and had landed a mediation process on the bemused Tessa which was clearly aimed at bringing the marriage to an end.

However, one could never be sure that the New Supply would turn up trumps. It was surely wise to have a first reserve, and Alex suspected that she herself had fulfilled that role for him. There had been an increasing warmth in Marcus's approaches early last year, by email, which had then cooled down again over a few walks together during the winter months. She wondered if his subsequent remoteness had, without her knowledge at the time, coincided with his taking possession of his new target sexually.

Once that conquest had been achieved, Alex could understand, in retrospect, that she would have immediately become redundant to him, even in terms of their platonic friendship. He was bound to have other dog carers in place, and he probably had other women eagerly volunteering to do his less rewarding research for him, just as she had done for the last six months. She grimaced to herself slightly, remembering the two Victorian novels of interminable length, convoluted narratives and almost indecipherable small print which she had waded through to summarise on his behalf.

She recalled the text message he had accidentally sent her from his mobile, three weeks ago, when she had been dog sitting Beano while he was away on one of his London days. What were the words again? 'Love U Sexy thanks for hier cant wait 2 C U.' When she had delivered Beano back to Marcus that evening, she had consciously chatted with him as usual, asking about how his meetings had gone, before gently pointing out the transit error to him. She was unsure as to whether he had flinched before brusquely acknowledging the mistake. He had added the explanation, 'I'm a man who must have secrets!' After that, she had hurriedly departed. Since then, the matter had not been mentioned between them. She glanced across at him uncertainly.

"May I ask how things are going with your.... your new relationship?"

He paused in response, eyeing her sharply as they followed Beano up past the brambles.

"Happy," he replied curtly. She kept her head down. There was a pause. "Does that distress you?" he added, in the same abrupt manner.

"No."

Her answer sounded a little uncertain, even to her. She repeated the response more firmly.

"No; I'm glad to think of you happy. It's been a very difficult time for you, what with your dad's death, playing mediator in the cathedral's political crises, separation from Tessa, selling your house, dividing your assets and finding a new place. It's good that you've come through to be happy, even so. But I suppose it's hard for me to understand why you need to eliminate our friendship because you've found a new, very significant one.

"When you first began to get in touch with me this time last year, I felt so very lucky to have another possible chance to be close to you. I had thought we would never see each other again and then, gradually, we were within arms' reach and then, after your separation from Tessa, finally able to walk and talk and be loving friends once more. I thought we had agreed back then that we would still be soul mates, and I do value your friendship very much."

"I'm not eliminating anyone," he replied swiftly. "I simply don't understand why you say that."

"Well, maybe it's just my problem," she commented quickly. "I feel as if I can't reach you at all, my love. It's as if I can't establish a feeling of safety for you with me. That is my failure, of course, not yours."

"Ah, but you're really saying that I act as if I want to keep my distance from you. So you are actually implying that I'm failing you. I don't feel easy with that. I don't feel comfortable with your analysis and metacognitive slant on things. I've had too much upheaval recently to want introspection. It's been a very challenging time for me, you know."

"Yes, darling; I can only try to imagine a bit what it must have been like; so much upheaval and pain. Maybe I'm remembering things wrongly here, but it seems to me that since you first started trying to get back into contact with me last spring, I've tried to take my cue from you. Once we were eventually able to meet, we've talked about your work, particularly the summaries of Carlton's last two novels, your moving preparations, cathedral politics, your next writing project, the reaction of Tessa and your kids and friends to your separation, and I honestly didn't think we were analysing. It has always been a joy for me to be with you, whatever we might be mulling over! D'you know, I still haven't lost that sharp lurch of excitement just before we meet!"

He made no reply. She plunged on nervously.

"I imagined that some of the incidental introspection along the way was at your instigation. But it's certainly true that I'm most interested in feelings because they seem to govern what we actually do or don't do, although we all seem to be blithely unconscious of that, most of the time. You pointed that fact out to me, long ago, expressed so beautifully by Matthew Arnold. D'you remember? You read me out a section of a long poem of his in your study once, though I forget its title now. The bit you read me was about the need to be connected to our inner world; a buried stream where 'what we mean we say, and what we want we know'...."

She tailed off as he appeared to be uninterested in the literary reference. She was presumably being irritatingly metacognitive again. She searched inwardly for an urgent shift of approach.

"Anyway, I expect your new happy relationship is taking creative energy to develop, especially in these hiatus times for you. Perhaps that excitement of a new shared world opening up means that the sort of friendship we thought we could rebuild is no longer of any relevance to you. You have a perfect right to discard it. I certainly won't fight you for its survival. What would be the point?"

There was a pause. He sighed, head turned slightly away from her.

"Here we are, focusing on me yet again. Why do you have a constant need to talk about our relationship and obsess about the nature of friendship? I really do have enough on my plate just now, as I've already pointed out, without additional issues to address."

She found herself completely lost for words. The silence between them expanded as they made their way towards the scrubby borders of the wood. She determined now to hold her tongue. It took her by surprise when he suddenly touched her shoulder lightly for a moment.

"Actually, perhaps I do have a need to destroy relationships," he conceded, head to one side. He suddenly swished at some brambly undergrowth ahead of him with his stick. "I've done it to other people in my life, here and there, over the years. I did it in my 20's to my best pal at Cambridge. Took up hours of his sympathy time and counselling advice, one evening, claiming I was heartbroken at a traumatic split up with Tessa, just as finals were approaching. (Like me, he was engaged to his childhood sweetheart, and we'd had many a deep and meaningful chat when either of us had run into girlfriend trouble.) He was immensely sympathetic, and in the end, I relented and told him I was having him on. He was furious, absolutely beside himself, and avoided me for the rest of our time there. It took years of me sending him a Christmas card regularly before finally he sent one back. I'm a loyal sort of bugger, you see. He was my best mate.

"So, on second thoughts, maybe it's inaccurate for me to say I need to destroy relationship. I think I sometimes need to smash up partnership rather than relationships. The moment I do it – when I see the shock in the other person's eyes – I feel as if I'm plugged into something real, something essential, a bit like St. Paul's light on the road to Damascus! It's as if confession liberates the soul from all artifice in one blinding, exhilarating moment. I can tire, sometimes, of watching a film of my life flickering past me. It's as if destroying the fabric of a partnership is a sort of compulsion in me which drives me to burst through the confines of the engagement."

"To be free of it, d'you think?"

There was a pause before he answered, "I don't know."

His tone had abruptly switched to slight boredom once more. "Here we are again!" he intoned. "Why should the attention be back on me? I feel under a spotlight with you, as if I'm being dissected. I don't want to be trapped on a psychiatrist's couch."

"Oh dear! I didn't think I was spot-lighting, honestly. I'm a bit surprised you say that. I've always sought for free space between us; at least that's what I thought I was doing.

"Somehow, though, it seems to me now that you are trying to break loose from that very space. Of course you're at liberty to do that as well, but is there really any need to make a bid for freedom if you're already unfettered? Have I somehow been binding the free space with briars for you, instead of fostering your 'hopes and desires'? If so, I feel sad and a bit helpless about that. Surely I'm focusing on me here when I'm telling you what I feel: sad. I've always prided myself – in a horribly arrogant way, I suppose – on not seeking to exert control over the people I love. I feel rather ashamed of myself if, actually, all that has been me deluding myself."

"So you're back to finding fault with me," he replied coldly. "I'm a failure who makes you sad and helpless, ashamed of your illusions. That's what you're actually saying, isn't it? You're just finding a clever way of turning it round and smudging it, to make it sound as if it's all about your responses rather than mine."

"Well, I am responsible for what I feel. I'm not blaming anyone else for it," Alex replied, trying to counter her own confusion. "I don't think I need to trawl through the reasons why I'm a bit mournful just now. I know why. But I'm not constantly sad. Other things in my life give me pleasure or upset me or worry me. But when I'm actually with you, my feelings will tend to be affected most by whether or not I feel both free and yet deeply attached to you, since it's that combination that I want during the times when I'm in your company.

"I used to call you my magician, remember? You're the only person I've ever known who filled me instantaneously with a sort of effervescent joy. It seems miraculous to me that you could make me feel happy and free and safe, all at the same time – and that you could continue to do so once we were only spending a couple of hours together a week, if that! If only we could both talk to the other about what each of us honestly feels now, then somehow, we might find our way back to a… a more open place. You used to say that you simply don't process any negative emotions you have, and you thought you'd get beyond them better if you did. If you don't want to do that, though, we needn't. It's your choice."

He was silent for several paces. Then he shrugged his shoulders slightly and sighed, "I can see that I should never have got back in touch with you again last year – it was clearly a mistake. You seem to want things to be how they were between us and that just isn't possible. You can't accept that it's different now."

She found it hard to follow this new twist in his line of thought, and flicked her hair back from her forehead with her fingers. Marcus was striding ahead of her now, trying to catch up with Beano who was bounding towards a footpath gate bordering the field.

"WA -IT …. WAAAAIIIT!" he commanded, projecting his voice towards Beano's furry rear. She caught up with him and they eventually passed through the entrance in the order he was specifying: she first, he next, then Beano. She waited until he was alongside her again. It was difficult to resume the conversation as he was now gazing to his left, towards the low lying hills. She eventually took up the thread.

"I do accept the difference, darling. You no longer want affection or intimacy between us, and I go along with that, though I do find mutual reserve difficult. You have found some use recently for my text reading or book packing or dog minding, which I offered because I wanted to provide it, without any pressure or even request from you. I always left the choice to you as to whether, how often and where we should meet, and to what purpose, because it honestly didn't matter to me, as long as we could both be together happily in kairos time when we did meet. Whatever your choice, I've enjoyed your company, I've valued your friendship and I love you. I never loved you in order to be loved back."

"But you told me recently that I was your 'Mont Blanc'. Your brother was killed on that mountain, for God's sake! You seem to imply I'm a dangerous, cold man, utterly indifferent to the pain of others who interact closely with me. How do you think it feels to be told that?" He glared across at her reproachfully.

"I can't remember the exact context of that conversation," Alex replied, pained by his expression. "But I remember you seemed to like the analogy of Mont Blanc then. We laughed about it, actually. You pointed out how lovely the high alpine pastures were, and I agreed. You referred me enthusiastically to a poem by Shelley with that title, which I did later look up and read.

"I think at the time you were talking about your capacity to close off all emotion if you needed to; to experience life through a sort of padding which muffled your ability to feel. I do remember that you said that other women have occasionally commented that you are a dangerous man. You yourself have told me that you are a man who must have secrets."

His eyes narrowed, and his voice was sharp in reply.

"I wish you wouldn't store up things I've said in the past and then use them against me in arguments. I am not required to be utterly consistent, you know. Feelings erupt, and dissolve and pass, as you have pointed out before now. If you want my feelings, I'm telling you. Your Mont Blanc comparison registers as an insult to me, and I resent it."

Alex felt perplexed and alarmed, struggling to keep her voice steady in reply.

"But I never thought of Mont Blanc as a murderous mountain because Bryan was killed climbing it. He loved climbing and respected the mountain's demands on climbers and the unexpected challenges of avalanches and rock falls. The mountain was beautiful to him. It is still beautiful to me. I don't see that something is devalued because there are dangers in engaging with it. It's once again as if you're rewriting things that I have said and putting them into a new context to twist them into hurtful remarks or deliberate lies of mine. I don't understand why you do that."

"Are you saying that I've been revisionist about your motivation before?" he queried. "I don't recall any such behaviour of mine."

"Well, you remember you claimed that I had lied about my contributing £5,000 to your fund raising, never letting you in on my plan, which meant you discovered about it only after tracing the source of the secret donation, much to your subsequent embarrassment. But actually, that's not how it was at all." Alex was trying to keep her voice gentle as she carried on with her version of events. "You'd kindly photographed the O'Rouke landscape of Mum's which I was planning to sell to get the money, and I used your digital photo as my initial approach to a dealer.

"A few months later, I went over to Belfast, to the Irish gallery, and negotiated with him. You knew all about it. Actually, you were impressed that I played a waiting game for almost a year, and eventually sold the painting for £13,000 instead of accepting the dealer's initial offer of £9,000. So your later accusation that I'd been deliberately underhand with you about the donation – even though you acknowledged it was a well intentioned deceit – was a complete reworking of the actual situation."

"Well, you know I don't claim to have a good memory."

"But this isn't just forgetting; it's revamping the whole incident with a sour twist of deceit and manipulation added in to my actions. Do you really think that's how I tend to behave?"

"Hmm... no," he responded vaguely. "I think you're usually rather open. I don't know. As a matter of fact, it's something I may have a habit of doing from time to time, misinterpreting things well after the event. I suppose I sometimes misread the situation in retrospect. It does cause confusion, I can see that, but at least it shows I'm trying to work things out. I'm simply not as skilled as you are at reading people on several levels at once. It isn't one of my strengths, I admit.

"Oh dear! I seem to have a sort of 'black fingers', rather than 'green' effect on my women, don't I? It's something I must look at one day; my urge to destroy members of the fair sex. They, au contraire, seem only too ready to cherish me!" He chuckled briefly, glancing up towards the silvery sky.

Alex found herself responding, "But.... but if you're embarking on a new loving relationship with a woman who really makes you happy, mightn't it be better to look at your urge to destroy before you get deeply involved with one another? I'm sure you don't want her to end up feeling devastated."

"So are you still intent on playing my couple-therapist then? Maybe that was one of the roles you provided for me privately in the past, through the odd marriage glitch with Tessa, but I don't need marriage guidance any longer, do I? I'm okay now. I'm a bachelor again. I've shed what I need to get rid of and I'm moving forward. You always said you wanted that for me, didn't you?"

He paused, glancing across at her pale face.

"We had some good times didn't we? You said you were happy with me back then."

"You were everything – everything to me," she replied softly.

"Well then, we did a lot for each other, didn't we? They were golden days."

"I learnt so much from you," she murmured eventually, eyes down. She was disappointed and yet relieved that he did not ask 'What?' Disappointed, since he evidently had no interest in the matter; relieved, because she did not know how she could have answered. It was unthinkable to reply that she had learnt so much about the nature of love from his contrasting position of anti love.

"There'll always be a part of you inside me here," she said quietly, her hand to her heart.

"Well, I grant you, we were certainly Unlike Poles in a state of attraction!"

She was silent for a few moments.

"Is that what it was to you, then; a brief encounter of electrons every so often? I remember it as much more than that: cor ad cor loquitur."

"I can't keep trying to live up to you," he replied briefly, eyes averted from her. "The 'language of the heart', 'unconditional love' 'attuned awareness', all that..... I mean, it sounds wonderful, but I eventually become exhausted trying to keep on that wave length."

"But you suddenly suggested to me not long ago that you felt you had used, abused and exploited me during our relationship. You sweetly even apologised for it, much to my consternation. If you honestly felt you have just used me, surely that can't have required much energy?"

"It isn't about using up energy; it's knowing that I'm not really on the starting blocks, as far as 'love' is concerned."

"But a loving relationship isn't a race, surely?" she replied earnestly. "Neither one of us can avoid surpassing the other in some ways, and lagging way behind, in others. I did struggle trying not to be cowed by your brilliant intellect at times, but then I'd say to myself, 'Well, he wouldn't want me to be genius, anyway.' It's pretty healthy to bring contrasting strengths into a relationship, since it allows each of us to learn more about what we lack and how we can shine. But perhaps I read it all wrong and you just think of us as User and Used up."

"As a matter of fact, I'm not thinking much about you and me at all," he replied coldly. "I've a considerable amount to deal with at this point in my life. And I've already said I dislike this sort of analysis since it achieves very little, to my mind. Shall we turn back? I have other commitments at four o'clock."

He was looking at her now. His voice was slightly softer, but there was still something ominous in his stance which scared her. She felt herself running out of energy somehow, almost as if the oxygen around her was becoming thinner. She nodded wordlessly, and they turned to retrace their steps. His last sentence had immediately indicated to her why he had selected a quarter to three for their meeting at Haydown this afternoon. The time limit meant that he could be sure to avoid any chance of genuine communication with her. There were some moments of silence before he spoke again.

"Tessa seems to be doing well, all in all. We were both tearful in our last dividing of spoils meeting. Splitting the family photos was difficult. We've had a lot of happy times together really, over the years. I shall never remarry, you know. There'll never be another Mrs. Hilton. I've told Tessa, 'I don't do families anymore.' I don't want the complications which arise from that sort of relationship. It's not her fault. It is simply that I've moved on.

"Nor do I wish to be in a relationship which may involve adultery. You're a married woman, after all, and you love your husband and your children. That isn't my scenario now. I'm refining my life, paring it down to the things I really want, cutting myself away from the trappings. It's a good feeling."

As Alex listened to him, she knew with certainty that this was the last time she would ever be in his company. One part of her was overcome with grief and loss at this thought, while the other knew that he was killing her softly with every word he spoke, and everything he left unsaid. If she wanted to live and thrive in the future, she knew she had to be away from him, and the sooner the better. The clash of these two responses left her feeling giddy, and she had to watch her step carefully over the uneven ground. She tried to tune back into his reflections.

"Tessa has been pretty good over these last months, I have to say. She was very supportive over Dad's death, even though we had only just separated then. It was hard for her, the funeral – a big Hilton family occasion, just when she and I had ceased to be a team within that family. My sisters and my mum were upset by our split up, actually. They wept to say goodbye to her."

"I thought you said your mum and sisters had always found Tessa difficult, though," Alex remarked in puzzlement, remembering a snippet of shared reflection from several years previously.

"No, they were all very fond of her, and sad to be losing her from the family after more than thirty years. It was a double whammy for them, really, as we were there to mourn the loss of my father at the funeral. I was in tears during the latter half of my address, standing there above them all, trying to steady myself by clinging on to the wooden surrounds of the pulpit for dear life. I choked up entirely just before the bit where I'd written that Dad was two days short of his sixtieth wedding anniversary. I simply couldn't speak for tears. I actually had to leave that whole sentence of mine out!

"I didn't even begin to say the first word of it. It had to remain unread! I went on to the sentence which followed it, and then I managed to regain my composure. I just about got through to the end. Everyone was very sweet to me afterwards, when I came down from the pulpit again. They were obviously very concerned about me, and they tried to comfort me but I still had tears running down my cheeks. We're a loyal clan, us Hiltons, you know. When things look bleak, we close ranks."

"Close ranks," repeated Alex, feeling dazed.

"I expect at least one of my sisters will keep in touch by email now and again with Tessa. It's a good sort of medium for that sort of maintenance of tricky connection, don't you think? Email has made such a difference to the way we build up networks; the potential combination of immediacy and a chosen degree of anonymity or even fantasy constitutes a communication revolution. I seriously think you and I would never have struck up a relationship at all if it wasn't for email. Don't you agree?"

"Well, I – um – I don't remember it being a key aspect at the beginning," she gulped. "We were in one another's company an awful lot of the week at work, weren't we? During all that time, we were most often talking one to one, face to face. But later – well, I suppose the emails became – er – more important between us...... once you had left the job and – well – from then on, we saw each other.... a lot less."

She found it hard to speak in complete sentences. It was very odd to be longing to be across the next two fields and onto the track which led to their cars, and yet to be wanting time to stop while she was still alongside him.

"Those little surprise packages of yours, though; those were such fun to open!"

She glanced over towards him in surprise. He seemed to be warmly nostalgic for a moment, a gentler look about his eyes.

"And even last time we met, when you were helping me with the book packing, you left that smoked salmon in my fridge and the delectable cheese and those other little treats. I remember thinking how lucky I was because there was almost nothing to eat in the house. Yet there I was feasting on luxurious little delicacies provided by my darling... darling.... Alex."

She caught her breath. He had faltered because he had forgotten 'Angel', his pet name for her, and had had to revert to her given name instead. They both knew it. There was a careful silence. She remembered saying to him once, 'One day, you won't even remember my name', which he had at that time vehemently denied. In this sudden memory lapse, he had ironically confirmed her fear by remembering her first name quite correctly.

"Oh dear! I've said something wrong again! Sharp sigh from Herself, small frown line curving above right eyebrow. Be quiet, Hilton, before you're told to see her in detention at quarter to four!"

"You can't get it wrong with me," she chorused, as she had so often said to him before, smiling across at him. "But you're welcome to meet me behind the bike shed whenever you want!"

It was a familiar code of humour between them and they both grinned at it. His face darkened again quickly though, and the amused tone had vanished with his next words.

"But I was the love of your life and I discarded you at Tessa's behest. You told me once that you were on a wheel of fire after that."

"My choice to feel that," Alex reminded him. "My feelings are my responsibility, not yours."

"So I haven't hurt Tessa or you or any other woman! It's just that they choose to feel wounded. How nice! I can do whatever I like then; carte blanche! I think you are a little too liberal at times, you know. If your philosophy were held more generally, the great forces which bind us to charitable behaviour and moral principle would crumble and anarchy would reign. Beano would like it, wouldn't you, Old Boy?"

Beano, intent on a thorough investigation of a rotting tree stump just ahead of them, did not raise his nose. For Alex, though, the turn of conversation was comforting. Marcus had often teased her tenderly for being an anarchist in the past, and this echo of laughter from their bygone days was a welcome relief.

"But you presuppose that our feelings will always lead us into chaotic behaviours," she replied, lightly parrying his thrust. "Perhaps if we excavated our feelings effectively and registered them accurately within ourselves, and also with the help of others, before we acted on them, we would feel more in tune with ourselves and thus be a lot nicer to everyone else. We wouldn't need a religious code to dictate those rules of niceness to us. I think that if we strip away our defensive responses and allow ourselves to be completely open and vulnerable, something strange happens; we become invulnerable. No one can really wound us because we are not engaging in defence."

"You are recommending Total Passivity then? So much for centuries of human initiative and progress!"

"Chosen vulnerability isn't the same as passivity; far from it! I think it would be very hard work to strip away defences which we've long believed are protection for our delicate egos. But if it was achievable, we wouldn't be emptied because all that remains would be Love."

"'Our almost-instinct almost true:'," he murmured.

She didn't recognise the quotation but smiled vaguely and nodded as if she did. It was evidently being used as a contradiction.

"Larkin," he added helpfully. "'An Arundel Tomb'. It won't do you know, my love, your philosophy. You disprove it by your own arguments earlier. You say you applied the principle of letting me free to do as I pleased in our relationship and now you are disappointed and saddened by me. So it seems that giving me freedom has allowed me to exploit you, for which I have apparently already apologised.

"Incidentally, I don't recall any such statement of mine, or any such apology. Actually," he continued, his tone gaining a little warmth, "I think you are determined to martyr yourself. Look at your dealings with men – a distant father, a brother who disappears in the Alps, a vanishing first husband, an anthropologist son who chooses to live on the other side of the world and to adopt a tongue and a culture totally foreign to ours, a second husband who is pretty far along the introverted scale..... and myself, of course, with my icy slopes and crackling crevasses.

"For someone who recommends the experience of giving up defences and engendering a warm fluffy world as a result, you seem to be extraordinarily attracted to cool operators and frosty environments. Have you really excavated your feelings to understand why you do that? Are you just a habitual rescuer of others because you won't face your own demons?"

Again, her response was immediate.

"Well, if I am – and I'm sure there's a lot of truth in that – it is your observations, and those of others who know me well, which might help me to begin to tackle that evasion." She continued with a rapidity which bordered on the passionate.

"How can we excavate unless we have someone else to sift through the layers with us? It's too scary to do it all alone, and we need the viewpoint of trusted others to help us to see ourselves more objectively. 'No man is an island' and all that. I suppose that's the value I see in shared analysis, which comes up incidentally from time to time in any truly intimate relationship, and benefits both people. I don't think it's the be all and end all of any connection between two companions of the heart, and it can certainly be overdone. It needs to come about naturally, in amongst both the dimness and the sparkle of regular shared experience."

She was suddenly aware that he was faintly repelled by her intensity. She added lamely, "But… but that's just my take on things of course."

She wondered about precisely who had been speaking up until she had faltered to a stop. For a few moments there had been a firmness and fluency about her pronouncements, in stark contrast to her earlier shakiness. She had no idea what she was saying until she had said it, and even then, she wasn't sure what was being affirmed, but somehow the affirmation itself was strengthening her.

In bygone days, he would have joined her at this point, plunging into an exhilarating exploration of ideas which would culminate in the apparent sharing of a breathtaking new conceptual free space together. She looked across at him as he stepped back to let her cross the stile onto the track first. His face was expressionless.

"Oh dear! I'm banging on again, aren't I?" she laughed, reaching her right foot down gingerly towards the wobbly wooden plank on the other side.

"At least Beano is intrigued!" he remarked, indicating Beano's pricked up ear as the terrier eagerly awaited permission to dive under the stile.

"I love that one ear up, one ear down look," she smiled, glancing back at Beano while Marcus joined her nimbly on the other side of the stile. She had more time to admire the enchanting canine pose as Beano stilled, alert for the command which would release him from 'STAY!' The wait seemed unexpectedly long, even to Alex.

"Come on, then!" was suddenly directed affectionately towards the dog, and once he was the other side, Beano was rewarded with a 'Good Boy!' and a noticeably loving fondle from his master. Marcus glanced up at her from his haunches as he drew Beano even closer to his side. He seemed keen, now, to explain the tenets of dog training.

"He has to learn the order of precedence; it is simply confusing for dogs, otherwise. They presuppose they are the leader of the pack and you have to demonstrate firmly to them who is boss. He used to be very attached to Tessa because she was the one who fed him. One evening, I came in late, opened the sitting room door and found him ensconced on her lap across the room from me. He growled. It was very quiet but it was most definitely a growl. I strode across the room, knocked him onto the floor and kicked him all the way through the room into the corridor and into the boot cupboard where he stayed for a good two hours. He never growled at me again. They need to learn who's top dog in the pack."

Her heartache seared even more intensely within her at this brief account of dog discipline. Marcus's pace seemed to be speeding up now that they were on the track which crossed the private airstrip. She noticed that he didn't glance to his right towards the field where, so often in the past, they had marvelled at the skylark's song, apparently coming from an empty sky, yet profuse and clear in its vibrant protection of its nest below. Lyrical dreaming days; a lost fantasy now. Would she ever be able to let go of it? What were those lines of Blake'?....

'But he who kisses the joy as it flies

Lives in Eternity's sunrise.'

She tried to catch up in order to walk beside him, but the track was deeply rutted and there was only room for single file along the firmer, raised section between the troughs. Beano had padded ahead of them, and Marcus was fumbling in his pocket for the lead.

She treasured this final chance to set her eyes on him, even with his back turned to her and the distance between them increasing as her pace slackened. She took in the sweet curl of his still dark hair into the nape of his neck, the straight back, the tailored shape of his body, the boyish swing of his walk, the general air of a compact man taking up additional space all around him.

There was something elemental about him: the glow of a child rigged up gleefully in adult dressing up clothes, deceiving no one, yet bewitching all. If he was her Peter Pan, she was well aware that her role as his Wendy was finished. Had he trapped his shadow and needed her simply to re attach it, as Wendy had Peter's? Was he a body who denied his soul, or a soul with no foot prints? How was it possible to feel so much love for him if he was, in fact, a man of no substance? Or was that very lack what gave him the essence of beauty? Although we might all be 'the stuff that dreams are made of', he seemed to be living that dream day by day. He was not as other men.

Ecce homo: behold the man!

He had reached the gap which accessed the bridle path. She knew at that moment that he had already gone; departed smoothly in his dark blue BMW long before it had even come into sight, parked at the muddy lay by opposite the farm pond.

EPILOGUE TWO

SUMMER 2008

Jenny's final walk with Ricky

Jenny felt surprised to find herself seated in the café this overcast Saturday morning. She was here because of a phone call from Ricky three days earlier, suggesting that they met up in the Portsmouth area for a chat. The phone invitation had been totally unexpected because the most recent email exchange between them, a few months before the call, had seemed to draw a final line in the sand.

Back then, Ricky had initiated matters by suddenly sending her a brief, lighthearted email, urging a meeting between them to renew their friendship, even if she might find it difficult to 'drop the image she had of him as a lying son of a bitch'. The detailed, heartfelt message she had sent in reply had elicited such a prime example of 'Word salad' (as Alex had labelled it) from Ricky that Jenny had abandoned trying to make any sense of it, other than that he had now given up on the idea of any sort of reunion.

Yet the subsequent, jaunty phone call from him, quite out of the blue, had made no reference at all to this bleak interchange over the airways, and Jenny had found herself drawn in to a rendezvous out of deep curiosity to see Ricky in the flesh one more time. She had brought part of the email exchange with her, in her handbag, as absolute proof to herself that there was no common ground between them. She took it out and let her eyes run through his last printed message, with the copy of her own missive laid out in all its earnest vulnerability beneath it.

'Subject: Ricky
Date: Tues, 27 May 2008

Thank you for your long and considered message in response to my recent suggestion for an encounter between us.

As you have reiterated, the sequence of past events have somewhat darkened your approach to me and consequently you feel that, under the circumstances, furthering of any deeper communication would inevitably result in a forthright rejection.

I also note that 'arrangements' as proposed wherein contact is maintained on a sparse basis does not constitute any sort of affiliation which would be of consequence. Therefore, it is with deep regret that I note this and subsequently will not endeavour to maintain contact with you. Any subsequent interaction would be solely in formal circumstances, if and when they transpire, the occurrence of which is unlikely.

'Ere I could
Give thee that parting kiss which I had sent
Betwixt two charming words,
And like the tyrannous breathing of the north
Shakes all our buds from growing...
Gone –flitted away,
Taken the stars from the night and the sun
From the day!
Gone, and a cloud in my heart.'
R'

'Jenny A< jallen23@mail.com> wrote:

I thought we had settled into a relationship of sorts. We've corresponded about twice a year and even met up once amicably. It is a fairly civilised way for exes to be. You haven't exactly been forthcoming over the last 10 years – it seems that only now when your relationship with Madeleine is rocky that you start to think back and feel some regrets! But I don't really know what you're after. Our relationship must have been foundering back in '98 for you to want to seduce Madeleine, knowing as you did my *feelings for you. (And we have never discussed your underlying reasons or feelings because you have never revealed them.)*

Actually, I don't think of you as a lying/cheating SOB. I was just so very very angry, hurt and humiliated that you obviously thought so little of me. You were able to discuss things, have your secrets and hide things from me for 18 months and yet never talk to me, your partner, about any of them. That anger of mine translated into wanting to cut your balls off – hurt YOU!

Now, 10 years later, I just feel very sad because I had been so wrong about someone I believed in. I thought back then that we had a shared relationship where we were at ease with one another after years of knowing one another well. I know we had problems but none of them were insurmountable, if we had discussed them together. Now I would never be able to trust you again or to believe in you as being honest and dependable and 'there for me' if we were in a close relationship again. How long would it last?

Now what? I can't offer more than a peripheral friendship. But I do think we have a shared history now that will always be part of 'us'. I don't know if you are after more. I dare say that when you meet another woman she would not be too pleased if you had a cosy relationship with an ex in the background, and might insist on my marching orders. Therefore you may want to finish our connection now. As I have often said, I am sad because of what might have been and I think you blew it all, not because of your infidelity but because you didn't know how to handle the subsequent fallout.

As always, J

She sighed and folded the page back up again, slipping it into a side pocket sewn in the lining of her bag. Soon afterwards, she looked up from her coffee towards the three people struggling to enter through the awkward gallery doors. Two women made their way over the threshold, nodding their thanks to the man who had helped them with the door before letting them go through first. She replaced her cup onto the saucer quickly and stood up when she saw the man was Ricky, his burly figure filling the cramped entrance space.

"Hello there!" he called jovially, striding over to embrace her, kissing her on one cheek and then nudging his face to the opposite side of hers, European style. She offered the second cheek just in time to have appeared comfortable with the greeting.

"Can I get you a coffee?" she asked, as he started to draw out a chair alongside hers.

"Yes, please! I'll have a latte."

He assembled himself on the café chair, leaning against the insubstantial aluminum back with more confidence than caution. He seemed totally relaxed, his bright eyes scanning the café space with proprietary ease. Jenny looked back at him from the dimly lit counter where she was standing to order the coffee. As always, she felt shaken, instantly altered somehow by his arrival, yet now finding herself engaged in the futile attempt to seem unaltered. His wide back was turned towards her, and from her waiting position she took in his longish hair, dark and somewhat greasy, lapping the collar of his corduroy Mattet. There was no trace of grey, no bald patch, but his hair was unkempt, flopping over his ears, casually stylish. He seemed to take up all the space around his table, and, indeed, around all the other empty tables. In the dim light of the café, he appeared somehow larger than life, self illuminated.

Completing her purchase, she walked carefully back towards him with the overfilled coffee cup, managing to place it in front of him without spilling any of it into the saucer. She seated herself again, glad to notice that she still had half of her own coffee left to drink.

"Well!" he said, smiling at her. "Isn't this just dandy!"

She nodded, smiling back with raised eyebrows, watching him closely as he continued speaking.

"It's been a long time since we sat in an art gallery café together – let me see now…God! This coffee's disgusting!"

He glared down at his cup, grimacing. "No blame to you, of course," he added rapidly. "T'anks for treating me." Jenny was silent.

"Any of yours in here?" he asked, waving a large hand towards the exhibition of paintings beyond the café.

"Yes. None of these are selected, though; you just donate them and they all go up."

"Oh, I'll have to see if I can spot yours later."

"I don't think you'd recognise my style anymore."
"Perhaps not, but I'd recognise the quality!"
Jenny snorted briefly.
"What? What's that sniff of derision for? I'd recognise artwork of yours anywhere."
His aquamarine eyes were fixed on her, a playful smile hovering around his lips. He looked for all the world like Gerard Depardieu, the cream open-necked shirt collar beneath his burnt sienna sweater whispering of summer in Provence, even in the pale light of a breezy Hampshire morning. She gathered herself in sharply.
"I've moved on a lot since you knew my artwork."
"Well, I'm sure you have. But I'll still hone in on your stuff. I'll show you, when we've swigged this abominable liquid!"
He shifted slightly on his chair, taking in the emptiness of the tabled area as he did so. He seemed momentarily to be searching for something, but then once more his gaze rested on her face. There was a short silence between them.
"I must say, you're looking very well," she burst out suddenly.
"I am very well! Why wouldn't I be?"
"No reason – I'm just saying, that's all."
There was another brief pause.
"Well, t'ank you. I make an effort to be easy on the eye."
" Not 't'ank you'…. 'thank you'!"
"Oh, hark at the English expert here! Just because you've got yourself a Southern English accent instead of that homely Derbyshire burr they all use up in the land of yer childhood."
"I never spoke with a burr. You're mixing me up with some other woman."
Jenny took another sip of her coffee, glancing at his face as she spoke. He twitched his mouth at her before remarking,
"As a matter of fact, the way the Irish speak is the true English pronunciation; th' way Shakespeare himself would have spoken."
Ricky grinned back at her.
"Th' way?!"
"Yes, th' way."
"It's 'the', not 'th' ! I can't imagine how on earth you taught English to the unfortunate Libyans with an accent like yours!"

"I adapt to my professional role, of course. I can do any number of accents as *The* occasion requires. I use my own when I feel at home. Unless the other person suddenly starts trying her best to make me feel uncomfortable......"

"You're saying you naturally feel at home with me?" Jenny stared at him hard. "Is that really true, Ricky?"

"Of course it is! We go back a long way, don't we? Why do you t'ink I sought you out again? And kept in touch by email and the odd wee mobile call when I could? You were never far from my mind, especially once I started working in Iran, where a man could find himself alone in his flat with a decided lack of female company and a need for some solo excitement.........."

He gave her a roguish grin, nudging her foot under the table. She couldn't hold herself back from a half smile, slightly flattered in spite of herself.

She lowered her voice to comment, "So I'm an occasional wank aid, am I?"

"More than occasional!"

"I see."

She didn't 'see', but couldn't think what else to say. It felt to her as if they were playing a game of 'Pass the Parcel' but with a multi wrapped explosive device at the core of the package.

They both sipped their coffee, almost in unison.

"So how long are you in England for this time?" she enquired evenly.

"No idea! I've finished one twelve week contract and I'm supposed to be taking up another in October, but I'm waiting for my visa to be renewed. The bureaucracy and red tape for entry into these various countries is unbelievable, and each time you return there after time in U.K., the whole ruddy process has to be repeated all over again."

"And where are you staying?"

Ricky's eyes took on a faraway look. "Oh, here and there – with the odd mate. I'm shacked up in the flat of a bloke called John in Southampton at the moment. You never met him. I'm squeezed onto his sofa."

"How does he feel about you being there?"

"Oh, he puts up with it!" replied Ricky airily. "I t'ink he'll probably be mightily relieved when I go, mind you."

Jenny said nothing to this. She was reflecting sadly that here lay the explanation for why he had kept in touch with her over all this time, with the odd unexpected call or brief email. He must have hoped that she might be prepared to supply him with a cosy base between contracts, if needed. It was not a new idea to her but nonetheless, the confirmation of its likelihood was painful. Presumably his Spanish supplier had provided home comforts as required over the last few years but there must always have been the need to keep other base suppliers in reserve, back in the ol' country, just in case primary supplier defaulted.

She recalled his proposal that they should meet, first mooted and turned down by her three months ago, and then repeated recently by phone. In the intervening time, a mutual friend, the only one who had sought to keep in touch with his old mate even in Spain, had reported to her that Ricky's relationship with her Spanish successor was now at an end. It had occurred to her to wonder how Madeleine was faring. The friend had responded that she seemed to be increasingly subject to bouts of depression.

Jenny had, after some angst but even more curiosity, accepted Ricky's second suggestion to meet, but she had specified exactly when and where. She was determined not to have him in her house or in any location where he could attempt to pounce. She was hoping that somehow, meeting him face to face would provide some sort of resolution for her, although she knew that this was extremely unlikely. The Langstone Art Gallery had seemed a neutral venue. She just wished she did not feel slightly sick.

She sought, floundering slightly, for a way to carry on their conversation.

"Have you been home to Ireland?"

"Not this time, because the Libyan Embassy still has my passport; I'm applying for another one but it hasn't come through yet. Most of us TEFOL teachers have a duplicate passport, and it's a good idea. Otherwise, you end up back here, homeless and stranded, rummaging t'rough rubbish bins and sleeping rough."

"Well, you certainly don't seem to have reached that point yet."

Jenny eyed up his clothing and his expensively casual tan leather shoes.

"I'll take that as a compliment!"

"Take it however you like."

The words came out rather more sharply than she had meant them to, but he didn't seem to register this, returning to her original question.

"I was in Ireland a year ago on another of these breaks between jobs. Not that I really have a base in Cork any more, but I saw the clan here and there – played tag wit' the granddaughter (she's seven now, for Gawd's sake!), caught up with one or two of the ol' fellas. I had a good awl blether wit' Martin; quite like old times. He was always the great talker."

Jenny summoned up a picture of Martin, Ricky's older brother, in her mind, without enthusiasm.

"I could never quite make Martin out," she reflected. "What about Damion? Did you see him?"

"Oh, I saw him all right! As usual, he hadn't a bloody word to say for himself. A crashing bore he's become! Mind you, he was never much crack at the best of times."

"Oh, I liked Damion. He's a kind, gentle man, but perceptive too."

"Well, surely I am the real gentleman of the family? I got the balance just right – not mouthy like Big Mart nor sullen like Wee Damion but the Main Man in the middle. I wasn't the favoured eldest nor the spoilt youngest! I was the pivotal brother, you might say."

"Damion isn't sullen." Jenny remembered Ricky's brother, a long time ago now, his hand resting briefly on her shoulder in the midst of drizzling Irish rain, just before she had slipped into the front passenger seat of the car. She had reached to kiss him on the cheek and he had spoken softly into her ear. 'He's not good enough for you,' he had whispered, and she had jerked her head away in surprise, embarrassed by what she took as an inappropriate approach to his older brother's woman. 'Not good for anyone who loves him,' Damion had continued rapidly, his head down towards her neck. 'Seven years at most, and then he's away off again. Watch out for yourself, Jenny.'

He had stepped back as she had seated herself in the car alongside Ricky. She had closed the car door very gently against Damion, but her quietness of movement had gone unnoticed because he had already turned his back to walk away from them both.

She had shrugged it off later, sitting close to Ricky as they drove back to Dublin after a cheerful fortnight of her being introduced to his town, his county and his people. She had enjoyed all the warmth of welcome she had received and had felt she was genuinely liked by his family, just as she liked them. Ricky had seemed pleased to bring his two worlds together so successfully and the only point of tension for her had been – at that last moment – Damion's unexpected mutterings. She had puzzled over them often, but not shared them with Ricky, fearing to cause further tension between the two brothers. She concluded again and again that Damion resented Ricky and had wanted to sew seeds of doubt in her mind about him. It was only recently that she had remembered the incident and had suddenly clicked that Damion had actually been giving her a vital warning which she had chosen to ignore. She sighed quietly. Ricky was still in full flow.

"........ t'inks he is superior but what has he ever done in his life except sit on his arse with the face of death on him ever since Ma passed away. Oh, sorry, now! Am I boring you or what? Was that a wee yawn?"

He leant towards her, peeping up at her with his head tilted. It flashed through her head that he probably knew this was one of his most enchanting poses.

"Do you want another coffee?" she asked quickly as a diversion, before remembering his verdict on the first cup.

"You must be joking! Come on now, point me towards the area where your stuff is and I'll prove to you that I'd know your style anywhere. No need to be bashful, is there? So! Shall we have a dekko, then? Is the show worth a glance?"

"Well, it's not a themed exhibition, as I said," replied Jenny, remaining seated despite Ricky's hand now being positioned on the back of her chair and poised to motion her upwards. "I haven't any idea what it's like; that's why I suggested meeting here, because I want to have a look. The gallery has just invited local artists to donate at least one piece of art work and then, at the end of this month, they have an event of some kind, and there's a lottery to have first pick of the donations, and then second, and so on. Every guest ends up with some specimen of artwork for the price of the entry ticket."

"Will you be at this shindig?"

"Oh no! The artists aren't invited to that. It'd be so awful watching one's picture being the last to be chosen. I only contributed something because of Sheila asking both me and Alex when we last had an Old Bags reunion; Sheila works here as a volunteer. But it seemed a good place for you and me to meet today because it's a long time since I've been here, and I just wanted to look at the general standard and how things were hung. I've got a list of all the contributing artists here."

She delved in her handbag briefly, grateful that the printout of their email exchange was tucked out of view. "And I'm perfectly happy about my name being among theirs – there's even a Sam Johnson, and Anne Ferguson has been extremely generous; she's donated three sketches. Anyone who knows their art will bid for one of those straight away. She sells in the hundreds now, even for pen and inks."

Jenny paused, hoping that Ricky would pick up on the names of artists whom they had once admired together. He didn't. There was a brief silence.

"Well, I'd bid for yours any day!"

"Don't be ridiculous! You don't even know which one it is."

"Oh, 'Don't be ridiculous!'" he mimicked, lips pursed. "You sound very properly English these days."

"And you sound very improperly Irish!" she retorted swiftly.

"How am I improper? I've told you already; I am the perfect gentleman."

"Hmpff! What exactly is your definition of a gentleman, may I ask?"

"A man who is honest and honourable, and a bit of a smoothie.... like me!"

"Honest and honourable?" she repeated incredulously, with a weak attempt at laughter in her voice.

"Well, I spoke the trut' about the coffee, didn't I? Come awn now, we'll glance at the walls and then have a walk by the sea, shall we? Could you drop me back at the train station once we've had ourselves a pub lunch? Are you up for that? Oh no! Wait! Don't tell me, you're far too busy to spare me t'ree more hours. You're all wrapped up in your running about the place with all these vital commitments to grandchildren and friends and lovers and God knows what."

Jenny decided to ignore the last part of his comment.

"Well, yes; I am probably busier than you are," she replied briskly. "But you've pointed out that you're just marking time before your visa comes through and you can start your next contract. I can't help it that you're in limbo and I'm not. This sort of mismatch is bound to occur when you walk out of a partnership and then drop in to check out the lie of the land, ten years later. We're strangers now, really, with no real concept of the other's life at all."

"Yours seems pretty okay to me. You're retired on a decent pension, you own your own place, kids and grandkids doing well, there's plenty of time for your art work and socialising with good mates living near you. You've got it really comfortable for yourself. More than I've achieved! I'm homeless in Hampshire, or drifting around, trading me skills in the English language like some sort of international pirate. Soon enough, anyhow, all us pirates will be totally out of a job because within a generation, everyone round the globe will speak English well enough for their needs, whatever their first languages might be."

"And then what?"

She couldn't resist asking him this, yet knew instantly that she wouldn't receive a straightforward reply. He would fog it somehow, as he always did.

"Then what?" he echoed, apparently puzzled.

"Well, what will you do when the pirate days are done; when you have to come ashore? Where is home for you? Where do you want to end up?"

"'Carpe diem' is my motto!" he exclaimed. "I'm an optimist! I genuinely believe that something good is always there for the asking, just round the corner."

"So is that why you left me? Because our relationship felt bad to you, and you were keen to sample something good just round the corner, with Madeleine in romantic Spain?"

He glanced across at her and lowered his voice slightly, his tone earnest.

"But you know I never left you in my heart. You'd be surprised at how often I thought of you. I really did feel bad about it all, and sort of not entitled to be happy when I knew you were alone and very pissed off with me. I was in a mess back then."

"But you're not now? It's all been sorted out, has it?"

"Well, yes, I suppose it has. I'm a free man now really, although, of course, I still have a sort of operational base in Spain. I love the place, you know; it really suits me! The people are so friendly and they are always up for fun and having a great time together. There's lots of amazing sights to see. I'd love to take you round Madrid, you know. It's a wonderful city!"

"Come on!" said Jenny, suddenly rising from her chair and leading the way up the three steps into the gallery corridor. She had felt that familiar surge of bewilderment beginning to invade her, and was anxious to regain control of herself. She had caught herself momentarily indulging in the warmth of Ricky's invitation and she was determined not to be left shivering again as a result.

She drew to a halt alongside a wall full of paintings and sketches, and glanced at her own framed painting's position to the top right of the wall, several paces away from where she was standing. Ricky strolled behind her, casting a nonchalant eye over the exhibits with that same slight smile on his lips.

"Well, am I to try to spot any of yours? Somewhere on this wall?" He seemed pleased to wheedle a new sort of game playing interlude between them. In spite of herself, Jenny was intrigued to discover whether he could indeed recognise her rendering of languishing tulips in sharp focus against the straight lines of a window sill, with the softened shapes of the outside foliage forming the background of the picture.

"Yes. Along here somewhere." She waved vaguely at the wall in front of her. She was careful not to glance in the direction of her painting and the two charcoal portrayals of chickens positioned alongside and beneath it. Ricky gazed from one end of the wall to the other.

"Well, I'd know those two aren't yours!" he commented, gesturing towards the charcoals with a dismissive wave.

"How do you know that?" she enquired, with interest.

"Well, you'd never do chicken drawings!" he announced grandly. She said nothing and he glanced at her briefly. "Well, certainly not as sketchily as that," he added. "Mebbe... Let me look more closely now; you might have done the tulips. Hang on!"

He wandered up along the wall one way, turned and then ambled back again, his eyes scanning the pictures once again as he passed them.

"I think perhaps it *is* the tulips. That's the sill of the kitchen window, isn't it, looking out onto the front garden? I like the way you've done it, contrasting the different levels of clarity and curves with straights. It's good." He nodded his approval. "How's the old Aga going these days?" he added unexpectedly.

"Just the same. I'm always grateful for it."

"Ah, and dear ol' Purdey! How he loved his corner place against the side of it! You could hear the purrs of him from outside in the garden. I hope there are Agas in Heaven for him; I'm sure there are."

Jenny was taken aback by the sudden intimacy of his memories.

"Hey ho, I think I'm about to be targeted!" he whispered genially, nudging a shoulder against her, and she glanced sideways to see one of the gallery managers, clipboard at the ready and evidently intent on launching an approach, moving rapidly towards them.

"I'll just pop to the loo," Jenny whispered, and turned back to escape along a dark corridor to the Ladies, grateful for a few quiet moments to compose herself.

When she returned, Ricky was standing in a commanding position, while the woman with short, wavy hair was talking up at his left profile enthusiastically. She had obviously identified him as a potential art collector and was leaning towards him, a flop of dark curls falling down over her forehead. As Jenny approached them, she realised that Ricky was being encouraged to buy a ticket for the Draw Night, and that he was playing along with the vendor, enjoying her misguided sales pitch. Jenny stood her distance, watching as the woman became even more animated, and Ricky smiled with feigned interest, head held back slightly, but attention directed downwards, since he towered above her. It was another minute or two before the conversation ended, he pocketed a flyer and then turned towards Jenny, beckoning her forward.

"Are we off, then?" he enquired cheerfully, and she nodded, stepping in front of him to lead the way out to the nearby car park.

Within a few minutes, they had arrived at the harbour and had embarked on the shore side walk. The sky above them was still more grey than white, and the sea was the colour of steel. It felt rather an appropriate backdrop to Jenny because she knew the high tide concealed the shallowness of the water, and somehow this seemed parallel to what she needed to remember about Ricky, metaphysically. As if to confirm her thoughts, she found him suddenly peering right up against her face.

"Is that glitter you have there on the top of your eyelids?"

She drew back momentarily. He sounded just like a curious three year old.

"Yes, it is. Don't you like it?"

"It's very fetching. Matches your shoes."

She glanced down at her sensible footwear. The brown leather was garnished with silvery toe caps and laces.

"Naturally!" she answered with a smile, as if she was proud of this coordination.

"I suppose this is where you bring all your fellas? You've never brought me here before."

"You've never asked me to," she answered promptly.

"Now, how would I have asked to come when I never knew this place existed?"

"So you like it?"

"It's great! It's so cutely scenic, isn't it? A quaint, old pub with benches outside, a picture-postcard mill, swans and ducks in the pond; it must be packed out wit' trippers in the sunshine. But I like it just like t'is now, wit' nobody around because it looks like rain. Sort of understated."

"So I'm nobody, am I?"

"Don't be obtuse! You know I meant 'nobody else'. Jeez, but you're a pedant, Jenny, you really are!"

They changed positions to go single file because the path was narrow between the marshes along one side of the pond, and the embankment to their right. Walking on in front of him, Jenny felt oddly wounded by his comment.

"Well, I feel like nobody to you, sometimes. That's what I mean," she explained. "Do you remember all those years ago when we used to say how lucky we were to have found each other and to have a second chance of happiness? I felt quite different back then."

"Did we say that? Oh yes! I remember now! We did, didn't we?"

He appeared faintly surprised. Jenny found his remark perplexing, struggling to put it into context of this meeting. There was a pause as she sought an explanation and voiced it out loud, without meaning to.

"It seems to me that you've lost any memory of what we were like together; of what you destroyed."

"Destroyed? Listen, *you* were the destructive one. Those letters you sent when you were mad at me! They practically ignited when I touched 'em! Any time I had a pain anywhere on my body for years after, I guessed you were sticking a pin in some wee effigy of me, a nasty gnome thing, wearing nothing but an Irish rugby shirt and exposing his horribly mangled genitalia to the world. It was scary, I can tell you! It's amazing me balls haven't shrivelled entirely and me willie is still in place – for the moment, anyway!"

"And do you have any idea *why* I was so angry?"

She had just about managed to suppress a smile at his words.

"None whatsoever," he replied blithely.

"No idea at all?"

She paused to allow him to come up to her, where the path had widened, and watched his untroubled expression as he responded.

"I don't analyse things for ever, the way you do. I live in the present because it's the best way. The past is over and done wit'! Just look at what remembering the past has done in Ireland over the years. Many, many lives lost because of hanging on to old woes. Best to travel without baggage."

"Like a pirate?"

"Indeed."

She could think of nothing further to say. All she could hear in his words was yet another dismissal of her. Why had he ever got in touch again if he was celebrating being a loner? Why ask her to Madrid? Why had she agreed to meet him at all? What else had she expected or hoped for? She felt numb somehow, and had to glance around her sharply to take in the reeds, the pebbled shore, the church spire in the distance. Soon she would leave him at the station and drive home and be safe. And sad.

They walked on in silence for a while. She was aware of him taking a surreptitious glance towards her now and again, but she kept her attention in front of her. Eventually, he broke into speech again.

"Oh, don't tell me, I've said the wrong thing again, haven't I? You can smack my tiny little rear end if you want to. I know I don't deserve it because I'll enjoy it so much but p'rhaps it'll give you some sense of retribution. Hell hath no fury like a woman scorned."

She glanced across at him, surprised.

"So you agree that you scorned me? Do you know what that feels like? Can you imagine it, if someone did it to you? I trusted you. I thought you felt about me what I felt about you. I thought we'd grow old together. Then you just plugged yourself into another woman and lied about that to me for over a year. And once you knew she was a safe bet, you just eliminated me and reinvented yourself in Spain with her. You even look Spanish, actually. And now I suppose you're about to reinvent yourself again, if things are all off with her."

"Everyone does some reinventing! We take on new projects, different jobs, new circumstances in life. You're reinvented now, aren't you? Just look at you! You're every inch the artist, these days, in that multicoloured ethnic yoke you're wearing, and yet there's that ginormous child seat in the back of your Nissan, to transport your treasured youngest grandchild. No talk of classrooms now, or exam results, or doing V.S.O. either, like in the old times. But so what? Who wants to be the same anyhow? It's better to adapt and to change wit' the times, not turn out to be a fossil...."

He suddenly started singing lustily, prancing along the path from one side to another.

"'Would you like to swing on a star?
Carry moonbeams home in a jar?

And be better off than you are?

Or would you rather be a mule!'"

She stood still and he overtook her, cavorting his way through the subsequent chorus. She couldn't help smiling. His movements were surprisingly graceful, despite their comic exaggeration and his formidable height.

"Should we turn back now?" she enquired, after a pause. "I think the pub fills up quite quickly. We might be best to get in before one o'clock."

"Aye, aye, Captain!"

He was now attempting to do a hornpipe, turning on the spot as she waited for his decision.

"Sing a sea shanty wit' me, me darlin'!" he commanded, hugging her to him briefly. Her nose was pressed up against the middle of his chest, momentarily. She pulled herself free a fraction later than she meant to.

"The tide's going down," she remarked sharply. "No sea shanties on an ebbing tide, as any decent pirate would know!"

"What about indecent pirates, though? We could ride the Spanish waves together indecently, give up respectable grandparenting, sail the seven seas! Or, if the lady prefers, we could walk sedately t'rough the fabulous art galleries of Madrid. All the world lies before you, yours for the taking. Just for now, though, we'll make for a Ploughman's Lunch in The Royal Oak, with a pint of Guinness to wash it down. How does that sound?"

"Oh, come on, then!"

She strode out ahead of him, glancing across towards the mud flats becoming exposed as the sea withdrew from the harbour. Her head felt muddled or was it muzzy? Did 'muddled' come from the word 'mud'? She didn't know, and suddenly a wave of helplessness seemed to overwhelm her and she found herself longing to be quietly planting rows of dwarf bean seedlings in her vegetable garden back home.

EPILOGUE THREE

SPRING 2010

Jenny and Alex

"So...... Are we any better than we were, say, three years ago; d'you think?"

"Oh yes! Definitely!" Jenny nodded vigorously, in affirmation of her own reply.

"And if Ricky contacted you again, and asked to meet up?"

"Um – well – I think I'd refuse; probably, I would. I know now it can't go anywhere. It always goes round in the same circle, doesn't it? Hope/ Imagined Connection/ Puzzlement/ Despair/ Head Done In / Hope. What would be the point? It'd only set me back, and things have felt much better this year. There's even the odd day now, when I actually don't think about him at all! He still haunts my dreams from time to time, and that might upset me for a few hours in the morning, but I can talk myself out of it."

"That cycle you mention – it's his cycle originally, you know, not yours – you've just taken it in because he landed it on you, to observe it working in you instead of in him. It has fancy names in the text books, the little sequence, but it's basically always the same sort of thing. He feels awful pain, and it's so severe it breaks through his non-feeling barrier and results in a moment of genuine self knowledge and even a brief connection with someone else. As soon as that happens, though, he is horrified by the threat of intimacy and retreats instantly back into defence. And that is where our Done In Heads come into the picture, because we get destabilised by their flickering closeness/ retreat/ closeness/ retreat."

Alex paused before asking,

"Do you still mourn the loss of the relationship?"

"Well, I know it wasn't a real relationship because it wasn't mutual. I was doing the involvement for us both, feeling my own, presupposing his. But I still don't understand why......."

There was a pause.

"Why what?" Alex enquired eventually.

"Why – er – why he couldn't tell me what was going wrong for him, or try to, anyway. Why couldn't he do what people usually do when a relationship runs into trouble somehow, and one of the two begins to feel frustrated and depressed about how things are going? I mean, isn't it obvious that they have got to look at it, poke at it, try to understand it, talk about it? Eventually, there'll surely be a way to work it through to some point of mutual understanding, however long it takes, whatever the outcome.

"That's what a relationship is about, isn't it? Being able to take the rough with the smooth, and keep the other person in the picture as it changes from smooth to rough and then into something else again. Why couldn't Ricky be bothered to do that? Instead, he just jacked the whole thing in and replaced it, without a second thought. Why wasn't it worth working at, from his point of view? And Joe had, long before, displayed precisely the same attitude. How could a man who seemed to love his children just wipe their significance out of his heart like that? How could these men simply give up on everything we had together, just as if it was a matter of changing your choice of breakfast cereal or washing powder? And why?"

Alex was silent for a moment. Jenny's words had disconcerted her. She negotiated the turn off from the main road carefully and changed into third gear as she reached the top of the rise. She was taking Jenny to a pub lunch before calling in to see the Artists' Cooperative's latest exhibition, where Jenny had, over the course of the last year, finally become comfortable to have her work on display among that of her new friends in the group. Then they planned to drop in at Hobbymarket before returning to Alex's house and subsequently journeying out in convoy for an early evening Old Bags' reunion. Elements of this agenda were fairly typical of how she and Jenny spent their time together when they met these days, once a month or so. Their notes and magazine cuttings about relationship dysfunction now lay undisturbed in a green shoe box behind Alex's piano. There was less talk of their past pains, and more of their art, crafts, children, grandchildren or friends. It had become unusual to be sharing a glimpse of the old despair.

"But, Jenny, you know the answer to that one, surely? These dear men of ours had come to be wired that way! Their thinking processes worked quite differently. Do you want them to be consistent about their loving feelings for those closest to them? You might as well expect a toddler to do a decent father of the bride speech! When we were in a so called relationship with them, we thought we were transmitting to them but actually, we were picking up the same airwaves we were sending out, simply bouncing back our loving of them onto us. It is the feeling of reaching out to them in love which so enhanced our lives alongside them, not the experience of interactive loving, created mutually by both partners. We simply gave them the benefit of the doubt, assuming that because it felt real and good to us, it must be reciprocated by them. But we were on a one way ticket to nowhere.

"Maybe we were easily fooled because of the difference in social background or academic level or Irishness versus Englishness – the 'otherness' of them. A disparity in class or professional environment or nationality or home language is bound to complicate matters; I expect a big age gap has the same effect. It would serve to protect a pretender, making relationship dysfunction much harder to identify, wouldn't it? We'd be likely to put down any perceived aberrations in the other person's interactions to the evident difference we already know about.

"Isn't it also possible, dear Jenny, that as time went on in our loving of our Narcissists, we began to suss them out a bit more astutely, even if we did not have the measure of them properly? Maybe we began to ask more searching questions here and there, and that felt threatening to them. They may have sensed that we were closing in on some sort of psychological mayhem within them which they were desperate to conceal. If they did sense it, surely they would want to get out of our orbit fast, and into a fresh encounter with an unquestioning, adoring new fan?

"You told me once that Ricky was fond of Keats, and that he'd left his copy of the poems at your house from when he lived with you, and had never asked for it back. Didn't you say that in that well thumbed, tatty volume, there was only one single bit of underlining, and that was somewhere in *Lamia*? Something about analysis being a turn-off?"

"Yes, that's right. I think the actual quotation is,
'Do not all charms fly
At the mere touch of cold philosophy?'
I suppose I should have sent the book back to him but I never did." Jenny shrugged, seeking to dismiss the suggestion of her own guilt.

"Well, perhaps Ricky underlined it because 'cold philosophy,' focused on him, – or could we call it 'detached observation' instead? – inevitably compelled him to replace his charm by harm, because he felt his cover might be blown at any moment?"

Alex was making this explanation up as she went along. "He had to do a preemptive strike in order to defend his shaky identity, although I very much doubt he would have been aware of what he was doing. He didn't know that you'd constantly rationalise even the oddest of his behaviour to yourself, always trying to make sense of the senseless, always trying to maintain your belief in him.

"Perhaps neither of us was willing to admit to ourselves that anything could be profoundly amiss with this soul mate of ours. We overrode our intuition whenever it tried to warn us. D'you know, I actually remember being with Marcus and feeling very weird; sort of spaced-out, once or twice, when I did that. I'd actually struggle to overcome some profound resistance of mine, as if I was breaking off some bit of myself, in my determination to stick to how I stubbornly wanted to experience things as genuine and right.

"We probably believed, you and I, that if, by any chance, there was something the matter with our beloved man, he would let us share it and give us a chance to support him through it. Little did we guess that if we had accidentally undermined him by our perplexity, he would employ a very different strategy to deal with our poised attunement: back off, duck out and replace! So, one day, much later on, we would find ourselves listening with growing alarm to his initial, awed appreciation of our replacement, with the hairs going up on the back of our necks, as you put it...."

Jenny smiled briefly at this, but continued to look troubled, glancing out towards the dark line of woods to their left. She half listened as Alex slipped into that old, familiar exposition mode, gathering momentum in a way Jenny remembered well from past conversations.

"We accept that our male toddlers, and I mean our sons in this instance, shared their worlds with us once, in the most joyfully loving and intimate of ways. We are resigned to the fact that now your Matt and his family are based in America for a while, and my Connor is in Japan permanently. We sensed this distance developing since they became teenagers, didn't we? The whole nature of our relationship with them is totally different now from how it was when they were very young. They don't share their orbits with us any more.

"Once, long ago, we were in on the excitement of their getting to the next level of *The Hobbit,* or we provided our delighted attention for their moon walking or skate boarding skills. We've had to learn to stand back, gradually, while still loving them as closely as ever. It isn't an unknown idea to us, then, is it, the need to love from a distance, as our children grow up and come to feel and think differently from how they once did. We knew it would change. We're both lucky to have one child each remaining in this country, still living within easy reach, even if the other is thousands of miles away.

"We'll have to learn that process of change and increasing distance all over again through loving and losing our grandsons, too, won't we?"

Jenny sighed and said nothing. Alex tried again.

"There is a difference, of course, between accepting this alteration in our relation to our kids, and their kids, in their turn, and really understanding that there will be no development from the toddler narcissistic stage with either Ricky or Marcus. The experience with our own sons may be painful, but we expected to have to go through this stepping back process with our own children and eventually, with their kids too. We saw it all happen, the other way on, in our own youth, didn't we? We expected that our parents would be able to let go of control over us, which, by and large, they did, given a few hiccups here and there. And there's always the chance that, like us, our offspring in their turn may remember their mums fondly, occasionally, and might even weep at our deaths in due course, as we have mourned the loss of our own parents."

Jenny's head was still lowered. Alex plunged on determinedly.

"Haven't we said to each other before, Jenny, that both you and I have been helped to get a bit saner by being so closely involved with Julie's Timmy and Bella's Little Jack, over the last four years? And you've had Matt's two kids to treasure, too, although I suppose that makes Matt's departure to America even more painful, to be losing contact with them as well.

"But anyway; grandchildren! I may be wrong, but I actually think being Jack's 'Bibi' is even more redemptive for me than being Mum to Connor and Paddy once was, because I can just enjoy Jack without so much of that ongoing responsibility which a parent has to shoulder.

"We've reflected often how having young sons, in particular, to bring up thirty years ago helped us when Joe and Liam departed. I expect that the mother/daughter relationship can be even closer in some ways, but we were talking about how cherishing small boys gave us a little egotist fantasy world to enter with them; they loved what we could supply and we loved supplying it. So even if we'd lost our supply-hungry lovers, we still had our fix of that spell binding, loving bond, only this time it was between our little demander son or grandson, and you or me, the very willing provider. I suppose it was a bit like being weaned off heroin by the use of methodin!

"Not being mum or grandmum to a daughter, I don't know if a little girl does the same rehabilitation job for us female wounded victims of Narcissist males, but I doubt it. A granddaughter probably provides the chance of a feminine magic all of its own, but I don't think that it works in a similarly restorative way as with a grandson. It all comes back to the particular emotional impact of cross gender intimacy, at whatever level and stage. At two intervals in our adult lives, you and I just connected ourselves, twice over, with delightful stuck male toddlers in disguise, and got ourselves right into their Wendy House games. Then we found ourselves marooned there, lost inside those shiny orange plastic sheet walls, while they raced over to the sandpit with little Phoebe Frilly Knickers. It's that simple for them, but for us, we grieve at full adult level about something that was just a kids' game to them."

"I understand what you're saying in my head, Alex. I just can't feel it any deeper down, to make it soothe the pain."

"Well, that's okay. You don't have to. Be nice to yourself. There are no rules about what you should be feeling. You're allowed to be hurt and sad."

"But I don't like the bruising ache I get sometimes! It grinds at me inwardly and, for as long as it's there, it destroys my peace of mind in the process. I know it's to do with this sense of turning out to be at crossed purposes in what seemed to be the most intimate and joyful of connections." Jenny sighed and hunched her shoulders.

There was a pause before Alex spoke again.

"I think Blake said something along the same lines:
'Joy and woe are woven fine.'"

She glanced across at Jenny in concern. The silence between them meant that she sought to expand on the quotation. "If we want to experience life to the full – and surely all artists want to do that, dear Jenny? – then we have to recognise that there's valuable payoff from the experience of fear and sadness; it protects us from the call to step out of our insulation. As long as we're sorrowful and scared, we can shield ourselves from attack and heartbreak because we're already bumping along the bottom of life, anyway. Sometimes we need that insulation to survive.

"But then again, in the cycle of life, maybe as it gets into spring and the weather warms up, there are more times when we feel more positive and we can move forward to forge connections again. Perhaps the primary restorative connection we need to make is between our head and our body. I suppose you and I have worked on that, haven't we, through doing our various Yoga classes and all those exercises about breathing and spine stretching and calming the mind? And then there are your dancing classes and even my body-pump sessions which might increase our awareness of our bodies, and reaffirm our integrated sense of Self in the process.

"And gradually, we begin to turn outwards again. We notice we are appreciating others, and making some sort of stronger link with them, despite the risks of being vulnerable to abandonment when we do. You and I have become super sensitive to any intuitive hunch of ours that we could be opening up to someone damaged who must cover this up by feigning appreciation or a desire for intimacy. We've learnt – for the time being at least! – that if that happens, we cut our losses and jump ship fast! But understanding the need to jump also means that we now hold all genuine others closer to our hearts than we ever did before, because the petty foibles of our preferences and prejudices drop away if we sense that any sort of genuine mutual connection could conceivably emerge, in whatever form.

"Once, I took that possibility for granted with everybody else I met, but I certainly don't now. We are so lucky if we can occasionally experience those moments of 'motiveless passion' (Krishnamurti's phrase) which we might get with someone or something else for an instant or, blessedly, for a lifetime. It doesn't matter what we are passionate about, as long as we can *feel*! Actually, there was another phrase, too – 'passive awareness' which, I think, sums it up even better because 'awareness' means we're tuned in for each opportunity in the present as it occurs, and 'passive' ...... well, I think it means we're not trying to control or engineer it. We're ready, I suppose."

"Ready for what?"

"Well, ready to face the unexpected, even if it hurts. Ready to postpone a response if that seems wisest. Ready to laugh and to celebrate when we can, and to mourn and to weep as long as we need to. Ready to find creative ways to redirect those passions of ours which need a different operational field from the one we've been stubbornly stuck in for so long. Readiness doesn't dissolve pain or guarantee joy, of course. But if it helps us to seize our chance to – um – to feel emotions alongside someone else who's doing that with us, too...... Well, it's the best we can aim for. It's as good as it gets.

"Think of those tragic phone calls which trapped people made from the twin towers on 9/11. None of those messages seemed to be saying, 'The key to the bank vault is on the third shelf of the wash room cabinet.' The ones I heard were all about sadness and love and reaching out one last time to the people closest to them. I honestly believe that what really matters most in life, what's most essential, are our closest two way relationships with other people."

"Hmpff! In that case, I'm just a catalogue of profound failure, as far as heterosexual relationships are concerned," sighed Jenny. "But it does console me to remember that my family history has three or four strong women in previous generations who ended up rearing large families single handedly, or forging their own way through their lives. One of them was a successful potter in the Thirties who did very well for herself – Alison Mayhew; her stuff is collectible now. And you've seen some of my great aunt Elsie Fraser's sculptures, haven't you? Hey, Alex – we're coming up to that Wellhead fountain to our left. Look! The water's flowing just as fast as ever, isn't it?"

"Wonder what it tastes like. D'you think it's drinkable?"

"Shall we?" There was a hint of goading in Jenny's voice.

They glanced at each other with amusement, and Alex swerved to the left, pulling up at a lay by just a little beyond the trough. She switched off the ignition and they flung open the car doors to step outside, exchanging a questioning glance at each other across the car roof. The noise of the splashing water reached them as they drew closer to the spring.

Jenny placed her cupped hand under the iron spout and scooped the water into her mouth, some droplets falling between her fingers and down her chin. Alex followed suit, and had just gulped down the little water she had caught when they both averted their eyes hastily from a passing car, followed immediately by a large van.

"Refreshing!" exclaimed Jenny, cupping her hand for another slurp of water.

"Thank you, old chap!" responded Alex, as she, too, reached forward, patting the carved lion's curly top.

"Odd idea to carve a lion at a place where horses are going to drink," she added, in passing. "And look, he's got windmills either side of him. Very strange!"

"He looks a kindly sort of lion, though," observed Jenny. She peered more closely at his face, supporting herself with one outstretched arm. "There's something – wait a minute – yes! There's something about his expression………"

"What?" Alex looked across at her intently, catching the mounting excitement in her tone.

"………I think it could be ……… 'motiveless passion'!"

"Aw, ya ratbag!"

Alex clutched for an extra scoop of water to flick at Jenny's face in retaliation for the barb, and promptly received a direct water hit back. A few moments later, another car went past but this time, it went unnoticed by both of them. The driver noticed them all right, though, and for some while afterwards, if thinking of surprising sights, he would recall the time he passed Wellhead fountain and saw two apparently respectable ladies of a certain age having a water fight, faces sopping, as if tears of laughter were running down their faces.

END PIECE

SUMMER 2010

Night time

"Bibi?   BIBI?"
"Yes, Snippy?"
"Is it morning yet?"
"No."
"Huh?"
"No – look! Can you see it's still dark out there, sweetie? We have to go back to sleep now, or you'll be very tired in the morning. And it's nursery school tomorrow morning which is hard work playing, isn't it? So you need all your sleep to make you strong to help out the teachers."

"But I don't want to go to nursery school in the morning. I want to stay here with you."

"And I want you here to play with me, Snippy, but we all have to go to work sometimes, don't we? And nursery school is your work. But it's only for the morning, and then Mummy will be back from her work and she'll collect you from nursery school and I think Lola and Sam are coming to play at your house. Then you can let your 'wild rumpus start'!"

"But I don't want to go to nursery school."

"But Miss Emily needs you at nursery school, doesn't she? And Miss Lorna, and Miss Sonia? The last thing Miss Sonia said when I collected you today was – d'you remember? 'Please come back in the morning, Jack; we really love it when you're here!'"

"But I want to stay here with you and play with my trains.

Maybe another parcel will come from ebayshop with blue track, and I want to see it come."

"That parcel came already, didn't it? And it had string round it and you pulled it and it came undone, remember? And do you remember what was in that parcel?"

"It was blue track! And there was dark blue track, too, and a funny sort of Edward and some people and some bridge bits and a broken train."

"But it didn't really matter about the broken train, did it? They were just extra bits which the man put in with the track. And do remember which one the broken train was?"

"Yes, it was Gordon but the wheels didn't go round properly. But Uncle Paddy and Auntie Anna bought me a new Gordon and his wheels do go round properly."

"And there was another parcel, before that, wasn't there, from the toy shop with the trains? There was Steam Thomas and Emily and Harvey and James. And the toy shop sent brown track because now they don't make blue track any more, do they? So we had to get blue track from eBay."

"But Neville was out of stop."

"Well, they'll make more Nevilles in the factory and then, one day, he'll come in another parcel from the toy shop, but we have to wait a bit. But now, we must try to go to sleep. Then Mummy will let you come again to Bibi and Pops's house, to stay the night. She wants you to sleep well so that you grow big and strong, and can go snowboarding like your daddy does. You have to eat good food and sleep lots if you want to get big and strong. We like our sleepovers every week, don't we? And tickling Pops when he wakes up? D'you want, 'Round and round the garden?'"

"Yes. I like you, Bibi."

"And I like you, Jackins."

"I don't want to go to sleep. How d'you know it's not morning, Bibi? Might be, it's morning?"

"Because it's still dark, Snippy; and 'cos no birds sing."

Recommended Reading

Section One

Books for readers interested in understanding human relationships

Bernstein, Albert J. *Emotional Vampires*, McGraw-Hill (New York, 2001)

Campbell, W. Keith. *When you Love a Man Who Loves Himself,* Sourcebooks, Inc. (Illinois, 2005)

Carter, Steven and Sokol, Julia. *Help! I'm in Love with a Narcissist*, M. Evans and Co. Inc.(New York, 2005)

Claxton, Guy. *The Wayward Mind,* Little, Brown (Great Britain, 2005)

Goleman, Daniel. *Emotional Intelligence,* Bloomsbury (London, 1996)

Goleman, Daniel. *Social Intelligence,* Bantam books (New York, 2006)

Halpern, Howard M. *How to Break your Addiction to a Person,* Bantam Books (USA, 1983)

Hare, Robert D. *Without Conscience,* The Guildford Press (New York and London, 1999)

Hirigoyen, Marie-France. *Stalking the Soul,* Helen Marx Books (New York, 2000)

Hotchkiss, Sandy. *Why is it Always about You?* Free Press (New York, 2002)

James, Oliver. *They Fxxx You Up,* Bloomsbury (London and Berlin, 2007)

Karpman, Steven. *Fairy tales and script drama Analysis*, Transactional Analysis Bulletin 7(26), 39-43 (USA, 1968)

Krishnamurti, J. *The First and Last Freedom,* Harper SanFrancisco (New York, 1975)

Krishnamurti, J. *Freedom, Love, and Action,* Shambhala Pocket Classics (Boston, 2001)

Lowen, Alexander. *Narcissism – Denial of the True Self*, Touchstone (USA, 1997)
Martinez-Lewi, Linda. *Freeing Yourself from the Narcissist in your Life,* Jeremy P. Tarcher/ Penguin (New York, 2008)
Moore, John D. *Confusing Love with Obsession*, Hazelden (Minnesota, 2004)
Payson, Eleanor D. *The Wizard of Oz and Other Narcissists,* Julian Day (Michigan, 2002)
Ramachandran, V. S. and Blakeslee, S. *Phantoms in the Brain*, Fourth Estate (London, 1999)
Scott Peck, M. *People of the Lie*, Simon and Schuster (New York and London, 1985)
Stern, Dr. Robin. *The Gaslight Effect*, Morgan Road Books (New York, 2007)
Stout, Martha. *The Sociopath Next Door,* Broadway Books (New York, 2005)
Walker, Anthony. *Siren's Dance,* Rodale Inc. (USA, 2003)
Zahn, Cynthia and Dibble, Kevin. *Narcissistic Lovers*, New Horizon Press (New Jersey, 2007)

Section Two

Books for students of social biology and the psychology of relationships

Brisch, Karl Heinz. *Treating Attachment Disorders*, The Guildford Press (New York, 2002)
Dawkins, Richard. *The Selfish Gene,* OUP (Oxford and New York, 1989)
Kalshed, Donald. *The Inner World of Trauma,* Routledge (London, 1996)
Karen, Robert. *Becoming Attached,* OUP (New York and Oxford, 1998)
Lachkar, Joan. *The Narcissist/Borderline Couple,* Brunner-Routledge (New York, 2004)
Masterson, J. F., ed. *The Personality Disorders Through the Lens of Attachment Theory and the Neurobiological Development of the Self*, Zeig, Tucker and Theisen, Inc. (Arizona, 2005)
Masterson, J. F., ed. *Psychotherapy of the Disorders of the Self*, Brunner/Mazel, Inc. (New York, 1989)
Masterson, J. F. and Lieberman, Anne R., eds. *A Therapist's Guide to the Personality Disorders,* Zeig, Tucker and Theisen, Inc. (Arizona, 2004)

Lightning Source UK Ltd.
Milton Keynes UK
UKOW050603270412

191574UK00001B/33/P